Easy Breathing

Natural Treatments for Asthma, Colds, Flu, Coughs, Allergies, Sinusitus

David Hoffmann
B.Sc., F.N.I.M.H.

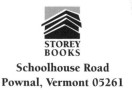
STOREY
BOOKS
Schoolhouse Road
Pownal, Vermont 05261

*The mission of Storey Communications is to serve our customers
by publishing practical information that encourages
personal independence in harmony with the environment.*

This publication is intended to provide educational information for
the reader on the covered subject. It is not intended to take the place
of personalized medical counseling, diagnosis, and treatment from a
medical doctor or other trained health professional.

Edited by Deborah Balmuth
Cover design by Meredith Maker
Cover art production and text design by Betty Kodela
Text production by Jennifer Jepson Smith
Illustration on page 3 by Alison Kolesar; all other illustrations by Charles Joslin,
  Beverly Duncan, Mallory Lake, Sarah Brill, and Brigita Fuhrmann
Indexed by Peggy Holloway

Printed in the United States by Versa Press
10 9 8 7 6 5 4 3 2 1

Library of Congress Cataloging-in-Publication Data

Hoffmann, David, 1951–
    Easy breathing: natural treatments for asthma, colds, flu, coughs, allergies, sinusitis /
David Hoffmann.
        p. cm. — (A Storey medicinal herb guide)
    Includes index.
    ISBN 1-58017-252-0
    1. Herbs — Therapeutic use.   2. Respiratory organs — Diseases — Alternative
treatment.   I. Title.   II. Medicinal herb guide
RC735.H47 H64 2000
616.2'0046 — dc21   00-038792

CONTENTS

1

HOW WE BREATHE

A remarkable thing happens when we breathe. Each breath that we take has been shared with all other human beings — in fact, with all other life on our planet. With respiration, we truly become one with nature. Trees and other growing things take in the carbon dioxide we exhale and replace it with life-giving oxygen. Through the circulation of gases in the atmosphere, the reality of the planetary whole reveals itself, with profound implications for all human life. This comprehensive vision underlies holistic healing as much as it does ecology. The anatomy and physiology of the respiratory system is a complex, beautiful embodiment of integration and wholeness.

Every minute, we breathe in and out 10 to 15 times. That adds up to nearly 25,000 breaths a day. Through breathing, the body extracts the oxygen it needs from the air and discharges carbon dioxide from the blood. The nearly 10,000 liters of air that we inhale daily consists mostly of oxygen and nitrogen. It also contains small amounts of other gases as well as floating bacteria, viruses, tobacco smoke, car exhaust, and other pollutants in the atmosphere.

Only one fifth of the air we breathe is oxygen, but this is the part that our bodies need for survival. Every cell in the body uses oxygen to extract the energy that's locked away in food. It's impossible to exaggerate the importance of oxygen. Many cells can survive briefly without it, but others need a constant supply. Brain cells die if they lack oxygen for more than a few minutes — and brain cells cannot be replaced.

The respiratory and circulatory systems supply the cells of the body with oxygen. This process is controlled by a part of the brain called the *medulla oblongata,* which regulates the breathing rhythm by integrating messages about blood composition with other signals.

THE WORKINGS OF THE RESPIRATORY SYSTEM

The lungs stretch from the trachea (also called the *windpipe*) to below the heart. They are safely encased within the thoracic cage and resemble a fine-grained sponge in texture. About 10 percent of the lungs is solid tissue; the rest is filled with air and blood. Because of this unique structure, the lungs can facilitate gas exchange — taking oxygen from the air and removing carbon dioxide from the blood — yet are strong enough to maintain their proper shape.

When we breathe, air is taken in through the nose and mouth and passes down the throat into the trachea. The air enters the lungs, where it travels into subdivisions called *bronchi*. The two main bronchi extend from the trachea into each lung. There, they divide into smaller bronchi, which divide again into many smaller bronchioles. The bronchioles divide into a network of about 3 million alveolar ducts. These ducts contain alveoli, which are commonly known as *air sacs.*

The Respiratory System

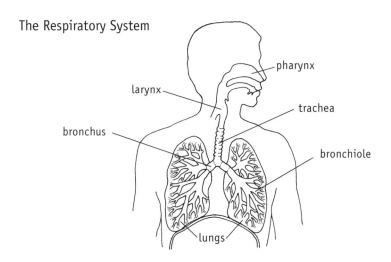

- pharynx
- larynx
- trachea
- bronchus
- bronchiole
- lungs

The Breathing Process

The movement of air into the lungs is controlled by the respiratory muscles of the thorax. These muscles, collectively called the *ventilatory apparatus*, include the diaphragm (the muscle that separates the chest and abdominal cavities) and the muscles that move the ribs. When the respiratory muscles contract, the chest enlarges like a bellows sucking in air. This is called *inhalation*. As the lungs fill with air, they expand automatically. They return to their resting size when we exhale.

The performance of the ventilatory apparatus is coordinated by specific nerve sites, called *respiratory centers*, that are located in the brain and neck. The respiratory centers respond to changes in blood levels of oxygen, carbon dioxide, and acid. Normal concentrations of these chemicals are maintained in arterial blood by changes in the breathing rate.

The outside of the lungs and the inside of the chest cavity are lined by membranes called the *pleurae*. The pleura surrounding the lungs is called the *visceral pleura*, and the pleura lining the chest cavity is called the *parietal pleura*. The space between the lungs and the inside of the chest cavity is called the *pleural space* or the *pleural cavity*. The pleural space is moistened with a fluid that lubricates the pleurae as they slide back and forth during ventilation. Normally, the pleural space contains only a small amount of fluid and is free of gas, blood, and other matter.

Gas exchange between our blood and the air we inhale takes place in the alveoli. The membrane that separates blood from air in the alveoli is very thin. In fact, it's about 50 times thinner than a sheet of tissue paper and has a surface area as large as a tennis court. Oxygen and nitrogen can pass easily through this membrane into the blood.

It takes just about a minute for the total blood volume of the body to pass through the lungs and only a fraction of a second for each red blood cell to pass through the capillary network. Gas exchange occurs almost instantaneously during this short period. The blood carries fresh oxygen throughout the body. When it returns to the alveoli, it deposits carbon dioxide and other gases, which leave the body in exhaled air.

The incredibly complex system that permits this continuous ebb and flow is what gives the body its life energy. Any physical problem that inhibits gas exchange will reduce the body's overall vitality and increase the risk for a variety of metabolic disorders.

THE HOLISTIC PERSPECTIVE ON DISEASE PREVENTION

Breathing problems do more than temporarily affect other organs and systems in the body. They can also cause chronic diseases. The reverse is true, too: For example, problems with the circulatory system can lead to lung problems. The condition of the digestive system is also important, since the lungs, bowels, kidneys, and skin share the task of removing wastes. If a problem develops in any of these organs, the body compensates by increasing the load on the others. The lungs can handle only a limited amount of wastes. So if, for example, the bowels aren't working properly and the lungs take on some of the burden, the lungs can also develop problems.

Many pathological changes in tissues can be prevented if the environment around the body's cells is always rich in oxygen. Two of the best measures for maintaining good health are getting regular exercise and promoting proper breathing. Balance and harmony, along with appropriate herbal treatments when necessary, are the keys to successful preventive medicine. We need a clear and free flow of energy through all aspects of our lives — physical, emotional, and spiritual. Proper breathing is just part of the equation.

A Whole-Body Approach to Breathing

It's impossible to separate the health and action of the lungs from the rest of our lives. People with healthy lifestyles are much more likely to have healthy lungs. Here are some of the most important factors in lung health:

- **Diet.** The foods we eat must ensure health and wholeness. The approaches people take to their diets depend on their specific health needs and personal preferences, which are always very important.
- **Body structure.** To maintain the body's integrity, we must address structural factors, such as any misalignment of the vertebrae. This may require the expertise of skilled practitioners. Exercise, of course, is critical to maintaining structural integrity.
- **Emotional needs.** A conscious and free-flowing emotional life is fundamental to inner harmony. This doesn't mean that everyone should get seriously involved in psychological counseling or other such practices, but it does mean that people should pay attention to their emotional needs.
- **Personal vision.** Mental factors are crucial. We are what we think! According to the bible, without vision, people will die.

Without a personal vision, life becomes a slow process of degeneration and decay. The emphasis must always be on *personal* vision rather than on a dogmatic belief system. Vision is an expression of the meaning in an individual's life. It must come from the core of his or her being.

- **Spirituality.** It's vital to be open to spirituality, which can take many forms: feeling uplifted by a sunset, being touched by poetry or art, believing in a religion, or simply taking joy in being alive.
- **Connection to nature.** In these times of ecological crisis and alienation from the natural world, it is most important to experience the embrace of nature. Using herbs is one way to do this. Other ways include walking in the woods or even hugging a tree. Smile!

THE KEYS TO RESPIRATORY HEALTH

As you can see, the best preventive strategy is to maintain a healthy lifestyle. Diet, exercise, and quality of life all have a profound effect on the health of the lungs. Our inner environments must be in harmony, and so must our outer environments. Polluted air will disrupt the ecology of the lungs just as it disrupts the ecology of forests. Air contaminated with chemicals, gases, and smoke should be avoided.

Specific Dangers to Avoid

This brings us to tobacco, which we'll discuss in more detail shortly. For now, keep in mind that smoking puts a wall of tar and ash between the individual and the world. A free ecological flow can't take place in the lungs of a smoker. Smoking can lead to an impressive array of problems, from bronchitis to cancer. It can also affect the rest of the body by diminishing oxygen supplied by the blood. If we want to heal ourselves and our world, quitting smoking is a good place to start. Even eating a whole-food diet and living in the country won't help if you smoke 20 cigarettes a day!

Specific dangers other than smoking should also be recognized and avoided. Infections are one such danger. The easiest way to avoid infections is to avoid contact with infectious agents. However, because this is often impossible, we need to maintain our natural defenses at peak levels. The body is capable of great feats of self-defense as long as we give it a balanced, vitamin-rich diet and follow a lifestyle that is healthy in thought, feeling, and action.

In this context, it's vital to curb the misuse of antibiotics. Although these drugs can save lives when used at the right time and in the right way, they can also weaken the body's innate defense systems. In addition, because these drugs have been used for a long time, highly resistant bacteria have developed and have made infections more and more difficult to treat. Over the past 30 years, doctors have seen alarming developments in microbial resistance. That's why it's so important to make the proper changes in lifestyle and to use herbal remedies when possible. The use of antibiotics can often be avoided when our bodies are strong.

In the following chapters, you will learn about how herbs can be used to boost the immune system, help maintain healthy respiratory functions, and assist the body in combating respiratory infections at an early stage.

THE MAIN THREATS
TO RESPIRATORY HEALTH

Many diseases commonly associated with the upper and lower respiratory systems can be prevented. Air quality is the key. If we avoid particulate air pollution and chemical irritants, like sulfur dioxide, many disabling conditions of the lungs will not develop. Smoking and inhaling secondhand smoke and urban pollution are important issues for practitioners as well as patients. Anyone concerned about the health of his or her lungs should become active in the environmental organization called Friends of the Earth.

Air pollutants such as photochemical smog, sulfur dioxide, and fine particles of coal dust affect the lungs in many ways. Some simply cause irritation and discomfort; others can cause illness or death. The lungs have a series of built-in mechanical and biological barriers that help keep harmful materials from entering the body, and specific defense mechanisms in the body can inactivate some disease-causing materials. Sometimes, though, the normal lung defenses and barriers do not work as well as they should.

Let's take a look at some of the risk factors for lung disease and the ways in which the body responds to them. Infections and other medical problems will also have a profound effect on how prone the respiratory system is to develop other problems.

However, these pathological causes are usually directly avoidable, as are many of the risk factors that derive from lifestyle choices.

TOBACCO: A LEADING HEALTH THREAT

Cigarette smoking, the single most preventable cause of death, is responsible for many life-threatening diseases, including lung cancer, emphysema, and heart disease. Tobacco smoke adversely affects many of the body's organs and systems. Every year, cigarette smoking directly causes an estimated 400,000 deaths. And every year, more deaths can be attributed to smoking than to fires, automobile crashes, alcohol, cocaine, heroin, AIDS, murders, and suicides combined. Passive smoke, often referred to as secondhand smoke, kills some 50,000 Americans each year, making it the third leading cause of preventable death in the United States. For every eight smokers who die as a result of smoking-related diseases, one nonsmoker dies of a disease related to secondhand smoke.

Cardiovascular Diseases

Smoking is responsible for 21 percent of all cases of fatal heart disease. It's a major risk factor for heart attacks and sudden cardiac death. In people who smoke a pack of cigarettes a day, the risk for heart attack is twice as great as in nonsmokers. In people who smoke two or more packs a day, the risk for heart attack is three times greater than in nonsmokers. Smoking is the principal cause of coronary heart disease — the most common cause of death in the United States — and increases risk for recurrence in people who have survived a heart attack.

Smoking is also an important cause of stroke and diseases of the blood vessels. It's the most powerful risk factor for atherosclerosis of the legs (also called *peripheral vascular disease*), which leads to leg pain, difficulty walking, gangrene, and sometimes, loss of limbs.

Cancer

Smoking is responsible for 32 percent of cancer deaths. It causes cancer of the lungs, oral cavity, pharynx, larynx, esophagus, pancreas, kidneys, bladder, and cervix. Recent evidence suggests that smoking is linked to cancer of the large intestine and to some forms of leukemia. Smoking causes nearly 90 percent of all lung and throat cancers. For many years, lung cancer has been the leading cause of cancer death in men, and it has surpassed breast cancer as the leading cancer killer among women. The risk for cancer increases with the amount and duration of smoking. Alcohol consumption is also a risk factor for cancer, and using alcohol and tobacco together greatly increases risk.

Respiratory Diseases

Smoking is responsible for 88 percent of deaths from chronic lung disease. It outweighs all other factors, including air pollution and occupational exposure to pollutants. Smoking harms the body's immune system and other defense mechanisms. The risk for respiratory infections, such as pneumonia and the flu, is higher in smokers than in nonsmokers. A recent study concluded that smoking increases susceptibility to the common cold. Cigarette smoking is a factor in up to 90 percent of cases of chronic bronchitis (sometimes called *smoker's cough*) in the United States, and it increases the likelihood of getting acute bacterial bronchitis. Air pollution also contributes to chronic bronchitis, as does working around dust or chemical fumes.

Effects on Pregnancy

Smoking directly affects the growth of the fetus. The more a mother smokes during pregnancy, the lower the weight of her newborn infant. Smoking increases the risk (by more than 50 percent in light smokers and by much more than 100 percent in heavy smokers) that a baby's weight at birth will be less than 2,500 g (about 5.5 pounds). Low-birthweight babies are more prone to adverse outcomes, including stillbirth, need for special treatment in neonatal intensive care units, and death in infancy. Smoking during pregnancy may also increase risk for miscarriage. Sudden infant death syndrome (SIDS) is more common in infants whose mothers smoked during pregnancy. Smoking also seems to decrease the quantity and quality of breast milk and may lead to early weaning.

Women who smoke during pregnancy also risk their own health. Abnormalities of the placenta and bleeding during pregnancy are more likely in women who smoke. The more a pregnant woman smokes, the greater her risks.

SPECIAL HAZARDS FOR WOMEN

In addition to increased risk of low-birthweight babies, there are other adverse outcomes of smoking that are unique to women. It's clear, for example, that smoking contributes to cancer of the cervix. Natural menopause occurs 1 to 2 years earlier in smokers than in nonsmokers. This may have unfavorable implications for women with conditions like coronary heart disease and osteoporosis. Smoking is also associated with an increased risk for menstrual disorders. Women who smoke are more likely than nonsmokers to have fertility problems. It's dangerous to smoke and use oral contraceptives — this increases the risk for heart attacks, stroke, and other vascular complications.

Gastrointestinal Effects

Smoking has been shown to harm all parts of the digestive system. It weakens the valve between the esophagus and the stomach, allowing stomach juices to *reflux,* or flow backward into the esophagus. Smoking also seems to promote the movement of bile salts from the intestine to the stomach, which makes the stomach juice more harmful. It may directly injure the esophagus, making it less able to resist further damage from refluxed material. Smoking seems to affect the liver, too, by changing the way the liver handles drugs and alcohol. Smoking contributes so strongly to digestive problems, in fact, that this alone is a good reason to quit. Peptic ulcer disease is more likely to occur in smokers than in nonsmokers. Ulcers heal more slowly in smokers and are more likely to recur. Current and former smokers have a higher risk for Crohn's disease than nonsmokers. Once current or former smokers contract Crohn's disease, they are more likely to have relapses, to require repeat surgery, and to need immunosuppressive treatment.

Effects on the Teeth and Gums

Tobacco contributes to oral cancer, but it also affects oral health in many other ways. In a recent study of Canadians 50 years of age and older, smokers were more likely than nonsmokers to have lost all of their natural teeth, to have teeth with decayed and filled root surfaces, and to have significant gum disease.

Whole-Body Damage from Smoking

It's hardly news that smoking is one of the greatest health risks Americans face. What people often don't realize is just how wide-ranging the dangers are. Here are just a few of the "surprising" conditions that can be caused by smoking:

- Decreased bone density of the lumbar spine and hip or osteoporosis, a bone-thinning disease that gives people, mainly women, a higher risk for bone fractures
- Graves' disease, a thyroid condition
- Reduced ability of the blood to carry oxygen to the cells of the body, which can lead to a plethora of problems, such as angina pectoris
- Increased heart rate and basal metabolic rate, which put extra strain on the heart

- Decreased blood flow through the small vessels of the skin, possibly leading to wrinkles and premature aging
- Cataracts

AIR POLLUTION

Air pollution occurs when gases, droplets, and particles reduce the quality of the air. In the city, air pollution may be caused by cars, buses, and airplanes as well as by industry and construction. In the country, air pollution may be caused by tractors plowing fields, trucks and cars driving on dirt or gravel roads, the operation of rock quarries, and smoke from wood and crop fires.

Ground-level ozone is the major significant air pollutant in most cities. It's created when engine and fuel gases that have already been released into the air interact in the presence of sunlight. Ozone levels increase in cities when the air is still, the sun is bright, and the temperature is warm. Ground-level ozone should not be confused with the "good" ozone that is miles up in the atmosphere and protects us from radiation.

If polluted air contains a lot of dust, fumes, smoke, gases, vapors, or mists, the risk for lung disease is increased. Poor ventilation, closed-in working areas, and heat also increase the risk.

Common Irritants in the Workplace

You should suspect a work-related illness if nose and throat problems occur when you are at work. Work-related exposures can cause bronchitis, asthma, and emphysema.

Following are some of the common workplace substances that can cause breathing problems and irritate the nose and throat, producing such coldlike symptoms as a runny nose or a scratchy throat:

- **Dust** from wood, cotton, coal, asbestos, silica, and talc is especially worrisome. Dust from cereal grains, coffee, pesticides, drug or enzyme powders, metals, and fiberglass can also hurt your lungs. Anyone working in the construction industry will be exposed, as will carpentry and agricultural workers. Even people working in the herb industry are often exposed to high levels of fine dust.

- **Fumes** from metals that are quickly heated and cooled release fine, solid particles into the air. Jobs that might involve such exposure include welding, smelting, pottery making, plastics manufacturing, and rubber operations.
- **Smoke** from burning organic materials contains various dusts, gases, and vapors, depending on what is burning. Firefighters are at special risk.
- **Gases** such as formaldehyde, ammonia, chlorine, sulfur dioxide, ozone, and nitrogen oxides can be dangerous. People working around chemical reactions or in jobs that use high heats, such as welding, brazing, smelting, oven drying, and furnace work, are at greatest risk.
- **Mists or sprays** from paints, lacquers, hair spray, pesticides, cleaning products, acids, oils, and solvents can be serious problems. People who may be affected range from hairstylists to artists using airbrushes.

Common Symptoms

Air pollution can irritate the eyes, throat, and lungs. Burning eyes, cough, and chest tightness are common symptoms of exposure to air pollution. However, responses to air pollution vary. Some people may notice symptoms; others may not. Because exercise requires faster, deeper breathing, it may increase symptoms. People with heart problems (like angina) or lung disease (like asthma or emphysema) may be very sensitive to air pollution.

For most healthy people, the symptoms of air pollution exposure go away as soon as the air quality improves. However, certain groups of people are more sensitive to air pollution than others. Children probably feel the effects of pollution at lower levels than adults do. They also experience more illness, such as bronchitis and earaches, in areas of high pollution than in areas with cleaner air. People with heart or lung disease also react more severely to polluted air. During times of heavy pollution, their conditions may worsen to the point that they must limit their activities or even seek additional medical care.

The Environmental Protection Agency (EPA) has established the Air Quality Index, until recently known as the Pollutant Standards Index (PSI), a uniform system of measuring pollution levels for the major air pollutants regulated under the Clean Air Act. The pollutants are particulate matter (soot, dust, particles), sulfur dioxide, carbon monoxide, nitrogen dioxide, and ozone. The index is reported as a number on a scale of 0 to 500 and is the air quality indicator cited in local newspaper or television reports. Index figures enable the public to determine whether air pollution levels in a particular location are good, moderate, unhealthful, or worse.

The most important number on this PSI scale is 100, since this number corresponds to the standard established under the Clean Air Act. A 0.14 ppm reading for sulfur dioxide or a 0.12 ppm reading for ozone would translate to an Air Quality Index level of 100. A level in excess of 100 indicates a pollutant reading in the unsatisfactory range. The complete scale is shown below.

POLLUTANT STANDARDS INDEX	
INDEX VALUES	DESCRIPTOR
0–50	Good
51–100	Moderate
101–150	Unhealthy for Sensitive Groups
151–200	Unhealthy
201–300	Very Unhealthy
301–500	Hazardous

INFECTIONS

Infections such as bronchitis and laryngitis are simply a part of living within Earth's biosphere. Humans are constantly in contact with vast numbers of bacteria, viruses, and fungi. The immune system has evolved so that this interaction is only occasionally a health problem. In fact, our well-being depends on maintaining a healthy and positive relationship with the range of organisms that live in and on our bodies (for example, the bacterial flora of the intestines and the microorganisms on the skin).

However, infections may occur when the body is exposed to pathogens that it can't fight. (Sometimes, even organisms that are usually nonpathogenic become a threat for some reason. The ubiquitous bacteria *Escherichia coli,* more commonly known as *E. coli,* is present in everyone as a normal member of the bacterial flora of the large intestine. If for some reason [and there are many reasons] the individual's immune system becomes weakened, *E. coli* may become pathogenic and cause intestinal problems.) If the immune response is compromised in some way, the ecological balance between the host (a person) and the various microbes changes.

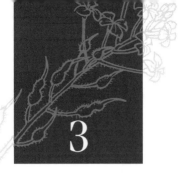

HOW HERBS CAN HELP

A lot of pharmaceutical research has been done to analyze the active constituents of herbs and find out how and why they work. However, a much older (and much more relevant) approach to categorizing herbs involves looking at the kinds of problems that can be treated with their help. In some cases, the action of an herb is caused by a specific chemical present in the herb. In others, it is caused by a complex synergistic interaction between various constituents of the plant.

The various kinds of herbs act in the following ways:

Adaptogen. Increases resistance and resilience to stress, enabling the body to adjust to a problem. Adaptogens seem to work by supporting the adrenal glands.

Alterative. Gradually restores proper functioning of the body, increasing health and vitality. Some alteratives support natural waste elimination through the kidneys, liver, lungs, or skin. Others stimulate digestive function or have antimicrobial properties, and others just work!

Anticatarrhal. Helps the body remove excess mucus in the sinuses and other areas. Mucus itself isn't a problem, but it can become one if too much is produced in response to an infection or as a way to remove excess carbohydrates from the body.

Anti-inflammatory. Soothes or reduces inflammation. These herbs work in many ways, but they don't usually inhibit the natural inflammatory reaction directly. Instead, they support the body as it is working.

Antimicrobial. Helps the body destroy or resist pathogenic microorganisms. Some antimicrobial herbs have antiseptic properties, but they generally work by strengthening the body's natural immunity.

Antispasmodic. Eases muscle cramps and helps relieve muscular tension. Many antispasmodics are also nervines, so they relieve psychological tension as well.

Astringent. Has a bracing action on mucous membranes, skin, and other tissue. Thanks to chemicals called *tannins,* astringents bind with protein molecules to reduce irritation and inflammation and create barriers against infections. These herbs are helpful in healing wounds and burns.

Bitter. Has a special role in preventive medicine. Bitter-tasting herbs trigger a sensory response in the central nervous system, and this response causes the intestine to release digestive hormones. Bitters are used to stimulate the appetite and the flow of digestive juices. They also aid the liver in detoxification, increase bile flow, and stimulate self-repair mechanisms in the gut.

Cardiac remedy. A general term for herbal remedies that have a beneficial effect on the heart. Some of the remedies in this group, like foxglove, are powerful cardioactive agents; others are gentler, safer herbs, like hawthorn and motherwort.

Carminative. Stimulates the digestive system, soothes the gut wall, reduces inflammation, eases gripping pains, and helps remove gas from the digestive tract.

Demulcent. Soothes and protects irritated or inflamed tissue. These herbs reduce irritation along the whole length of the bowel, reduce sensitivity to potentially corrosive gastric acids, and help prevent diarrhea. They also reduce the muscle spasms that lead to colic and bronchial tension, which causes coughing.

Diaphoretic. Promotes perspiration, helping the skin eliminate wastes from the body. Some diaphoretics produce observable sweat, and others aid normal perspiration. They often promote dilation of surface capillaries, improving circulation. They support the work of the kidneys by increasing the cleansing that occurs through the skin.

Diuretic. Increases the production and elimination of urine. In herbal medicine, with its ancient traditions, the term is often applied to herbs that have a beneficial action on the urinary system as a whole. Diuretics help the body eliminate waste and support the process of inner cleansing.

Emmenagogue. Stimulates menstrual flow and activity. The term is also applied to remedies that normalize and tone the female reproductive system.

Expectorant. Stimulates removal of mucus from the lungs and acts as a tonic for the respiratory system. Stimulating expectorants "irritate" the bronchioles, causing expulsion of material. Relaxing expectorants soothe bronchial spasms and loosen mucus secretions, relieving dry, irritating coughs.

Hepatic. Aids the liver by toning and strengthening and, in some cases, increasing the flow of bile. These herbs are very important because the liver's role in the body is fundamental.

Hypotensive. Decreases abnormally high blood pressure.

Laxative. Stimulates bowel movements. Long-term use of laxatives should be avoided; diet, general health, and stress levels should all be closely considered when constipation persists.

Nervine. Helps the nervous system. Nervine tonics strengthen and restore the nervous system, nervine relaxants ease anxiety and tension by soothing both body and mind, and nervine stimulants directly encourage nerve activity.

Rubefacient. Generates a localized increase in blood flow when applied to the skin, encouraging healing, cleansing, and nourishment. These herbs are often used to ease the pain and swelling of arthritic joints.

Tonic. Nurtures and invigorates. Tonics truly are gifts from nature to a suffering humanity. To ask how they work is to ask how life itself works!

Vulnerary. Promotes wound healing. Usually describes herbs that heal skin lesions. Vulneraries also work for internal wounds, like stomach ulcers.

HERBS FOR FIGHTING INFECTIONS

Medicinal herbs have a critical role in battling respiratory infection such as bronchitis. Many herbal remedies have antimicrobial reputations, but we must remember that they don't always achieve the desired results. This is why antibiotics are so important. Antibiotics can save lives when used the right way; the scourge of epidemic infectious disease has largely disappeared from the Western world because of antibiotics. Smallpox, for example, has been completely eradicated — a truly miraculous achievement. Herbal therapy can't always deal with severe acute infections, especially in people with weakened immune systems. Serious infections often require antibiotic treatments. As a dedicated herbalist who recognizes the limitations of herbal therapy, I celebrate the existence of antibiotics. After all, the role of the healer is to alleviate suffering, not to promote a belief system.

Antimicrobial Actions

Herbal medicine has limitations, but it still has a lot to offer. In fact, herbal treatments contribute a great deal to the fight against infection. For example:

- Herbs can boost the immune response and help the body rid itself of pathogens.
- Herbs can directly kill an offending organism. For this to be effective, however, some constituent in the herb must be able to reach the site of infection, and this is difficult to achieve.

- Herbs tone and strengthen tissues, organs, and entire body systems that are the focus of an infection.
- Herbs can facilitate recuperation from infections and help the body deal with antibiotics.

Even though many herbs can be used to help the body destroy or resist pathogenic microorganisms, it's a mistake to talk about herbal remedies as being *antibiotic* because this term literally means "antilife."

With herbal remedies, the body may be able to strengthen its own resistance to infectious organisms and ward off an illness. Although some plant remedies contain chemicals that are strongly antiseptic or poisonous to certain harmful organisms, herbs generally work by aiding the natural immune processes. Many plants with antimicrobial effects also act as anti-inflammatory, antiviral, and antiparasitic agents by strengthening the body's overall immunity. Antibiotic drugs are often essential, but not as often as people may think. The body can benefit from supportive and preventive help that bypasses the need for chemical intervention in an emergency.

Examples of Antimicrobials

Each system in the body responds best to different herbal remedies. Because of the nature of infections and the body's immune response to them, a general systemic treatment is always appropriate, even though it may be combined with specific local remedies. For example:

- **Respiratory system.** The main remedies are echinacea, wild indigo, and myrrh. Other helpful herbs include aniseed, balsam of Peru, clove, elecampane, and thyme, which have various expectorant effects.
- **Circulatory system.** Garlic is appropriate because it has beneficial effects on the cardiovascular system in general.
- **Digestive system.** Many remedies that contain volatile oil and some digestive bitters have antimicrobial effects in the

intestines. Herbs to consider include echinacea, garlic, gentian, marigold, myrrh, sage, and wormwood.

- **Urinary system.** Some of the urinary antimicrobial remedies are too powerful to use when there's a possibility of kidney disease. In general, though, effective remedies include bearberry, echinacea, eucalyptus, juniper berries, and yarrow.
- **Reproductive system.** Echinacea, garlic, and southernwood can be used, as can the urinary antimicrobials.
- **Muscular and skeletal systems.** Echinacea and wild indigo are a good basis for treatment.
- **Nervous system.** St.-John's-wort or pasqueflower, given in combination with nervines and other antimicrobials, will help the body cope with intransigent infections that can affect the nervous system.
- **The skin.** Many antimicrobial herbs can be used on the skin. A wash of garlic, marjoram, rosemary, or thyme can be very effective. Myrrh is one of the strongest external remedies.

ANTIMICROBIAL HERBS

Nature has been very generous in supplying us with antimicrobial herbs. These include:

Aniseed	Elecampane	Osha	Wild indigo
Balsam of Peru	Eucalyptus	Peppermint	Wormwood
Bearberry	Garlic	Rosemary	Yarrow
Calendula	Gentian	Rue	
Caraway	Goldenseal	St.-John's-wort	
Cayenne	Juniper	Sage	
Clove	Marjoram	Southernwood	
Coriander	Myrrh	Thyme	
Echinacea	Olive	Usnea	

ECHINACEA: HOW ONE ANTIMICROBIAL HERB WORKS

As antimicrobials, herbs seem to work in two broad ways. The main way is by stimulating the body's immune system (myrrh does this, for example). A second way is by directly killing microorganisms (herbs that do this, such as garlic, thyme, and eucalyptus, are usually rich in volatile oils). It's not always clear how herbs work, but extensive research on herbal medicines is currently underway. Let's look at some of the research that's been done on one particular herb, echinacea.

Research Results

Most of the research on echinacea is laboratory based. (As is often the case with plants, few clinical trials have been done.) It has been suggested that the primary antimicrobial constituents in echinacea are the echinacoside glycosides. However, many other biologically active substances are present, and evidence shows that they work synergistically. For example, echinacea contains polysaccharides, which are antiviral and have immune-stimulating properties. Other constituents have been shown to have good antitumor, bacteriostatic, and anesthetic activities.

Here's what some of the research has shown:

- Glycosides from the roots of echinacea have mild activity against *Streptococcus* species and *Staphylococcus aureus*. Echinacoside is the most active compound; about 6 mg is equivalent to 1 unit of penicillin.
- Echinacea tincture is able to reduce the growth and reproduction rates of *Trichomonas vaginalis*, a common pathogen of the reproductive system.
- Echinacea was found to be effective in preventing the recurrence of *Candida albicans* infection, or thrush.

- Echinacea seems to prevent infection and to repair tissue damaged by infection, partly by inhibiting the activity of the enzyme hyaluronidase.
- Purified polysaccharides prepared from echinacea activate the body's macrophage-mediated defense system. This is important because the large macrophages initiate the destruction of pathogens and cancer cells. Also, the macrophages are instrumental in the production and secretion of interleukin-1 and B cells.
- Researchers from the United States Department of Agriculture have discovered that echinacea has a constituent that inhibits tumors.

In summary, echinacea, like many other herbs, primarily affects the way the immune system functions. This means that it helps prevent and cure various pathogenic infections.

A GENERAL APPROACH TO TREATING INFECTION

Because many herbs stimulate the immune system in similar ways, we can make some generalizations about treatment. However, the details vary with the nature of the disease, the person using the herbs, and any other medications that are being used at the same time. The following are some guidelines for selecting appropriate herbs.

- Choose herbs that are best suited for the particular site of the infection. For example, elecampane can be used for lung infections; pleurisy root can be used for infections of the pleural membranes.
- Consider your age and general condition. As a rule, people who are very young, very old, or very ill should use gentler herbs. For example, coltsfoot is very mild and therefore is a

good expectorant for children, whereas the stronger blood-root is a good expectorant for adults.

- Always use tonic remedies along with antimicrobial herbs. For example, use mullein for lung infections and osha for throat infections.
- Support the body by using diaphoretics, which promote perspiration and help the body deal with any fever that accompanies the infection. Elderflower, ginger, and yarrow are all examples.
- Alleviate symptomatic discomfort when necessary. The specifics will vary with each infection.
- Use herbs to support antibiotic therapy. There's no reason to discontinue phytotherapy while treatment with antibiotics is underway. Once a course of antibiotics has been completed, herbs may be used to speed recovery, prevent recurrence of infection, and prevent secondary problems caused by the temporarily weakened immune system.
- Focus on general nutrition, and enlist the help of herbal tonics. For example, use bitters to safely stimulate normal metabolism; use gentle diuretics and hepatics to help support elimination; and use tonics specific for the area of the body that is the site of infection and causes the most discomfort.

COMMON RESPIRATORY
CONDITIONS AND
TREATMENTS

Different conditions of the digestive system produce common processes, symptoms, and general experiences. Knowing herbal approaches that will address these general patterns helps the herbalist treat a specific disease.

In this chapter, we will discuss the most common respiratory ailments, their symptoms and causes, and how herbs may be used to help ease the symptoms and address the root causes. The ailments are arranged in an order that builds progressive knowledge about herbs as you proceed through the chapter. We consider the expectorant herbs first and the ailments that benefit from this group of herbs, including coughs, bronchitis, and asthma. Then we consider the anticatarrhal herbs and the conditions that benefit from these herbs, including colds, flu, hay fever, sinusitis, sore throat, and tonsillitis. As I have said, the basic philosophy of herbalism is to look at the whole person, not just the specific ailment. I encourage you to read this chapter from beginning to end to fully understand how your particular symptoms might be related to more than one ailment. In this way, you will learn about how the interrelatedness of the various functions and problems of the respiratory system and how herbs may be used to address more than one aspect of this system.

EXPECTORANTS

Expectorants are herbs that help the body remove excess mucus from the lungs and airways. However, the term *expectorant* is very badly used and misdefined and is often used to mean a remedy that "does something" for the respiratory system. Herbal expectorants can actually have a range of properties, including acting as a tonic, a stimulant, or a relaxant.

Tonics

The expectorant tonics have a beneficial effect on lung tissue and overall function. These herbs, also known as *pulmonaries,* help the body remove excess mucus from the lungs. Important expectorant tonics include elecampane, mullein, and coltsfoot. The different indications for each of these herbs can be found in chapter 5. To generalize, elecampane has stimulating expectorant effects, and mullein is more of a relaxing expectorant. Coltsfoot is the best of the three for children.

Stimulating Expectorants

The stimulating expectorants act in many different ways, and it is not always clear how a specific remedy is working. It is thought that some irritate the bronchioles, stimulating the expulsion of mucus from the lungs. Others help liquefy mucus so that it can be cleared from the lungs by coughing. The fine hairs of the ciliated epithelium, which line the bronchiole tubes, move sputum upward from the lungs. Expectorants can make this transport easier by reducing the viscosity of the sputum.

> ### Spices as Expectorants
>
> Spices promote expectoration by stimulating the salivary and gastric glands and by increasing the production and reducing the viscosity of bronchial secretions. This explains why spicy foods help ease chronic bronchitis and also why bland foods tend to exacerbate it.

Most stimulating expectorants contain alkaloids, saponins, or volatile oils. Here's how they work:

- **Alkaloid-based action.** For example, in ipecacuanha, the major component is an alkaloid called *emetine*, an emetic that increases gastric secretions and induces nausea. The alkaloid also affects the bronchial mucosa, further increasing gastric secretion. Some other expectorants work this way and at high doses can cause vomiting.
- **Saponin-based action.** *Primula officinalis*, an expectorant common in Europe, contains 5 to 10 percent saponin and 0.25 percent volatile oil in its roots. It can be used for all forms of chronic bronchitis, especially "simple" coughs that last a long time and are characterized by inadequate expectoration. The action of the saponins here is not clearly understood. It may be based on reflex mechanisms induced through gastric stimulation that's mediated by the vagus nerve. The effect is much less marked than that of ipecacuanha.

THE EXPECTORANT HERBS

Stimulating Expectorants		Relaxing Expectorants	
Balm of Gilead	Squill	Aniseed	Lobelia
Balsam of Tolu	Sweet violet	Coltsfoot	Lungwort
Bloodroot		Comfrey	Marsh mallow
Cowslip		Goldenseal	Pleurisy root
Daisy		Grindelia	Skunk cabbage
Elecampane		Hyssop	Sundew
Horehound		Iceland moss	Thuja
Ipecacuanha		Irish moss	Thyme
Senega		Licorice	Wild cherry

Relaxing Expectorants

The relaxing expectorants would seem to act also by reflex, but here the effect is to soothe bronchial spasm and loosen mucus secretions. This loosening occurs when the expectorant produces a thinner mucus, then lifts the stickier mucus up from below. For this reason, the relaxing expectorants are particularly useful for dry, irritating coughs.

Some of the relaxing expectorants are anti-inflammatory and mildly antimicrobial because of their volatile oil content, while others are muscle-relaxing antispasmodics. The actions of this latter group are due to alkaloids or volatile oils.

COUGHS

Should coughs be soothed, stimulated, or suppressed? A cough is an important diagnostic signal from the body, and in most cases you should not simply suppress it. Any longstanding or intransigent cough should receive professional attention.

Home treatment is safe and effective for minor coughs that are of short duration or are associated with mild infections. Even in these cases, it's always best to seek skilled advice. You should focus on the underlying cause of the cough because it might not be enough to treat just the cough itself.

WHAT CAUSES A COUGH?

Coughing is a reflex response to anything blocking the airways. Usually this is mucus secreted by membranes lining the respiratory tract. Such mucus secretions help to protect the respiratory tract from any kind of irritant, trapping and flushing out smoke particles, bacteria, and viruses. Any cough that lasts more than a few days, does not respond to treatment, or produces blood should be investigated further because it may be a sign of serious organic disease.

Simple Cough Elixir

The honey in this recipe has antimicrobial properties and also acts as an expectorant.

1 large onion
Organic honey

To make: Slice the onion into rings and put the rings in a deep bowl. Cover with honey and let stand overnight. In the morning, strain the honey-onion juice mixture, reserving the mixture and discarding the onion slices.

To use: Take 1 teaspoon of the mixture four or five times a day.

Herbal Cough Tea

This formula includes some of the herbs traditionally associated with cough suppressants.

1 part coltsfoot
1 part marsh mallow leaf
1 part hyssop
1 part licorice

To make: Combine the dried herbs and make an infusion as directed on page 113.

To use: Drink as often as needed until symptoms subside.

Expectorant remedies will help expel phlegm from the lungs, soothe irritation, and reduce the cough reflex. When a cough is dry and irritating, it's best to use a demulcent, such as marsh mallow leaves, to soothe the inflamed membranes. Mullein, which is stronger than marsh mallow, may be used for coughs in adults.

Coughs caused by acute inflammatory conditions of the respiratory system are primarily treated with mucilage-rich herbs, like marsh mallow leaves. The stimulating, saponin-containing expectorants are not appropriate in all cases because they are best for subacute or chronic bronchitis, which requires active expectoration.

Seek Medical Attention for a Chronic Cough

A chronic cough lasts for at least several weeks. It should always be checked by a physician, especially if you notice any of the following:

- The phlegm is thick, yellow, or green.
- Your temperature is higher than 101°F (38°C).
- You're losing weight.
- You're having drenching sweats at night.
- You're coughing up blood.

Could Heartburn Be the Cause?

Occasionally, stomach acids back up into the throat, a condition known as *acid reflux*. This relatively common and unpleasant problem occurs when the lower esophageal sphincter, the muscular valve connecting the esophagus with the stomach, weakens and allows stomach acids to escape. The main symptom is heartburn, but acid reflux may cause coughing as well.

Dietary and lifestyle choices contribute to this condition. Certain foods and beverages, including chocolate, peppermint, fried or fatty foods, coffee, and alcohol, may weaken the lower esophageal sphincter. Cigarette smoking also relaxes the valve. Hiatal hernia, a structural weakness of the diaphragm, is a major cause, and obesity and pregnancy may also be responsible.

Heartburn is the main symptom of acid reflux. It feels like a burning pain that begins behind the breastbone and moves upward to the neck and throat. It might feel as though food is coming back into the mouth, leaving an acid or bitter taste. This might last as long as 2 hours and is often worse after eating. Lying down or bending over can trigger heartburn. Heartburn pain can be mistaken for the pain associated with heart disease or a heart attack, but there are differences. In heart disease, exercise may aggravate pain and rest may relieve it. Heartburn pain is less likely to be associated with physical activity.

Herbs to Consider for Heartburn–Related Cough

Any specific treatment plan or list of remedies for a condition reflects herbal wisdom and experience gained through history. Lifestyle and dietary changes are effective at relieving the symptoms for most people. Treatment aims at decreasing the amount of reflux or reducing damage to the lining of the esophagus from refluxed materials. In this section, we'll look first at the relevant

---

Tincture Formula for Heartburn

This formula combines demulcent and anti-inflammatory herbs to soothe and reduce inflammation.

2 parts marsh mallow root
1 part calendula
1 part chamomile

To make: Combine dried herbs with alcohol to make a tincture, as described on page 115.
To use: Take 5 ml of the tincture three times daily. Supplement with a cold infusion of marsh mallow root sipped slowly throughout the day to minimize symptomatic discomfort.

herbs, followed by other options to consider. These remedies should not be considered a substitute for a balanced prescription that considers the needs of the particular individual.

Possible treatments for heartburn and related cough include:

- Demulcent herbs, such as marsh mallow leaves, which soothe and coat the tissue of the esophagus, insulating it from acidic stomach contents
- Anti-inflammatories, such as chamomile, lemon balm, and calendula, which reduce any localized mucosal reaction
- Wound-healing vulneraries, like comfrey and calendula, which aid the natural healing process of damaged esophageal tissues
- Astringents, like meadowsweet, which lessen any minor local bleeding
- Carminatives, like chamomile, which may be needed if there is a more general disruption of the digestive process

> **CAUTION!**
>
> Bitters may be harmful for people suffering from heartburn because they stimulate the secretion of stomach acid.

Simple Steps to Relieve Heartburn Symptoms

The following lifestyle changes will reduce most of the symptomatic discomfort of heartburn while you are treating the underlying problem:

- Raise the head of the bed. This reduces heartburn by allowing gravity to minimize the reflux of stomach contents into the esophagus.
- Avoid stooping or wearing tight clothes; both put excessive pressure on the abdomen.
- Avoid foods and beverages that can weaken the lower esophageal sphincter. These include chocolate, peppermint, fatty foods, coffee, and alcohol. Foods and beverages that can irritate a damaged esophageal lining, such as citrus fruits and juices, tomato products, and pepper, should also be avoided.

- At mealtime, decrease the size of your portions. Eat meals at least 2 to 3 hours before bedtime. This may reduce acid reflux because the acid in your stomach will decrease and your stomach will partially empty before you lie down.
- Lose weight if necessary. This often helps relieve symptoms.
- Give up cigarettes; smoking weakens the lower esophageal sphincter.
- Do your best to deal with stress and anxiety.
- Use antacids, which neutralize acid in the esophagus and stomach and can help stop heartburn. Long-term use of these drugs should be avoided, however, because they may cause diarrhea, altered calcium metabolism, and the buildup of magnesium in the body. Excessive amounts of magnesium can be harmful for people with kidney disease.

BRONCHITIS

Bronchitis is an acute or chronic inflammation of the mucus lining of the bronchial tubes, the main airways that carry air from the trachea to the lungs. The inflammation may be caused by a viral or bacterial infection, by smoking, or by the inhalation of chemical pollutants or dust. The types of bacteria that cause acute bronchitis include *Streptococcus pneumoniae* and *Haemophilus influenzae*. Acute viral bronchitis usually clears up without treatment.

Bronchitis is extremely common. From July 1994 to June 1995, more than 5 million Americans developed acute bronchitis. In 1994, the American Lung Association estimated that about 14 million Americans were affected by chronic bronchitis. This makes chronic bronchitis the seventh-ranking chronic condition in the United States.

When the cells of the bronchial lining are irritated beyond a certain point, tiny hairs called *cilia*, which normally trap and eliminate pollutants, stop functioning. Mucus clogs the air passages, and irritation increases. In response, even more mucus develops, causing the cough that is characteristic of bronchitis.

The pain associated with bronchitis may be related to the swelling of the mucous membrane in the trachea. Other symptoms include persistent coughing, aching associated with fever, and mucus secretions. People with bronchitis are tired and often find it difficult to move. This desire to be inactive is caused by fatigue resulting from a lack of oxygen.

Treatment Approaches

Complications from a cold or the flu may lead to acute bronchitis, which can be treated by getting bed rest, drinking plenty of fluids, and staying inside during damp, cold weather. Acute bacterial bronchitis usually lasts about 1 week and is accompanied by a cough that produces thick green or yellow mucus. This type of bronchitis may occur after a cold in a healthy person or may flare up in a person with chronic bronchitis.

People who have series of acute bronchitis attacks, smoke heavily, or breathe polluted air may develop chronic bronchitis. Because this condition can be life threatening, it should receive professional medical attention regardless of its underlying causes. It's not uncommon for people with chronic bronchitis to cough up mucus nearly every day for months or years.

Because the approaches to acute and chronic bronchitis are so different, I'll discuss them separately.

ACUTE BRONCHITIS

Acute bronchitis is often accompanied by fever, usually lasts for a few days, and is characterized by a harsh and painful cough. Short-lived bouts of acute bronchitis often follow a severe cold and may follow or accompany the flu. Acute bronchitis usually originates from a viral infection in the upper respiratory tract and later spreads to the lungs.

The disorder typically lasts for about 10 days. Severe cases may cause general malaise and chest pain. The cough is very dry at first but becomes easier and less painful as the lungs produce additional mucus in response to the infection, lubricating the bronchi. Persistent fever suggests pneumonia. Although acute bronchitis is usually mild, it may be serious in debilitated people and people with chronic lung or heart disease.

Acute bronchitis usually occurs when viruses get into the bronchial tree, attacking the lining and causing damage. The body's immune response to the viruses leads to more swelling and increased mucus production. Even after the viruses are killed, it takes time to repair the damage, and an intransigent cough with accompanying wheezing persists. Things that aggravate the damage, like cigarette smoking, will lengthen the healing time.

Sometimes the cough from acute bronchitis lasts for several weeks or months. It takes this much time for the bronchial lining to heal. However, the cough may be a sign of other problems. For example, acute bronchitis can be confused with asthma. If you continue to wheeze and cough, especially at night or when you're active, you may have mild asthma. Also, pneumonia and acute bronchitis sometimes have similar symptoms. If you have a high fever, feel very sick and weak, and have a persistent cough, you should visit the doctor.

WHEN TO SEE A DOCTOR

Bronchitis is occasionally caused by acid coming up from the stomach and dripping into the lungs during sleep. If your cough continues and is accompanied by a bad-tasting fluid in your mouth, you should see your doctor. A doctor should also be consulted if:

- The mucus is greenish yellow and thick rather than gray and watery.
- The chest pains become severe.
- The cough lasts more than 1 month.
- The illness is accompanied by a fever.
- You're coughing up blood.
- You have difficulty breathing only when you lie down.
- Your feet swell.

The best defense against acute bronchitis is to avoid smoking. Smoking damages the bronchial tree, makes it easier for viruses to cause infections, and slows healing. After avoidance of cigarettes, the following regimen is the most effective way to deal with acute bronchitis:

- Avoid fatigue by getting adequate rest.
- Stay indoors when the weather is cold, windy, and damp.
- Drink large amounts of fluids to help keep chest mucus liquefied.
- Avoid use of cough suppressants.

Herbs to Consider for Acute Bronchitis

Any specific treatment plan or list of remedies for a condition reflects herbal wisdom and experience gained through history — we are blessed with many options that have been found and developed over the centuries. There is usually more than one "correct" way of doing something. The remedies given should not be considered a substitute for a balanced prescription that considers the needs of a particular person.

The use of soothing, relaxing expectorants in conjunction with antimicrobials is often the key to successful herbal treatment. Keep in mind that every individual (and every condition) is different. Although all of these herbs will be effective in some cases, they aren't appropriate all the time. Herbal treatments that may be considered for acute bronchitis include the following:

- Tonic pulmonaries, like mullein or elecampane, are not crucial if the problem isn't recurrent, but it's always a good idea to tone.
- Stimulating or relaxing expectorants can be used, depending on the indications.
- Antispasmodic herbs, like wild cherry bark, may be helpful when coughing is troublesome.
- Antimicrobials, like garlic, can deal with any infection and help protect against secondary infections.

Soothing Cough Tea

A soothing combination that is indicated for a dry, unproductive cough.

> 1 part mullein
> 1 part coltsfoot
> 1 part marsh mallow leaf
> 1 part aniseed

To make: Using dried herbs, make an infusion using 2 teaspoons of herbal mixture for every 1 cup (240 ml) of boiling water, and infuse for 20 minutes. See page 113 for full instructions.

To use: Drink hot several times a day.

Congestion Relief Tea

A gently stimulating herb tea that will help loosen congestion in the lungs.

> 1 part cowslip
> 1 part thyme
> 1 part coltsfoot

To make: Using dried herbs, make an infusion by adding 2 teaspoons of herb mixture for every 1 cup (240 ml) of boiling water. Infuse for 20 minutes. See full instructions on page 113.

To use: Drink hot three times a day.

HERB CHOICES FOR ACUTE BRONCHITIS

Aniseed

Balm of Gilead

Bloodroot

Coltsfoot

Cowslip

Elecampane

Fenugreek

Garlic

Goldenseal

Horehound

Hyssop

Irish moss

Licorice

Lobelia

Lungwort

Mullein

Osha

Plantain

Pleurisy root

Skunk
  cabbage

Sundew

Thyme

Vervain

Violet

Five-Herb Tincture for Acute Bronchitis

A strong immune-system booster for fighting infection.

1 part elecampane

1 part horehound

1 part coltsfoot

1 part goldenseal

1 part echinacea

To make: Combine dried or fresh herbs with alcohol as instructed on page 115.

To use: Take 5 ml of the combination tincture three times a day. Supplement with a daily dose of garlic (raw or in capsule form).

External Remedies for Acute Bronchitis

Plants that are rich in volatile oils (also known as essential oils) are often used for steam inhalations, which can sometimes halt the development of a cold or even the flu. When an infection is already established, inhalations will loosen mucus and clear the sinuses.

To make a steam inhalation with fresh or dried herbs: Place a handful of chamomile flowers in a bowl and pour boiling water over them. Drape a towel around your head to create a "tent" as you lean over the bowl and trap the steam. Breathe in deeply.

Other herbs that may be used for inhalation include thyme, eucalyptus, and marjoram.

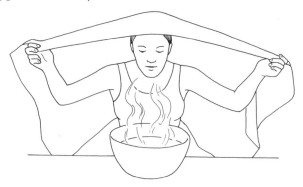

To make a steam inhalation with essential oils: You may prefer to use pure essential oils rather than the herb itself. The oil of dwarf pine needles *(Pinus pumilio)* is the most common recommendation, but others can help, too. Other recommendations include oil of thyme, eucalyptus, peppermint, or Asian mint. It's best to use oils at the onset of symptoms. Put three to five drops of oil in a bowl. Add boiling water, and inhale the steam for 5 to 10 minutes. The vapor may be irritating, so keep your eyes closed.

Massage with essential oils: You may find massaging the essential oils directly onto the chest, back, or neck to be helpful. This allows the active ingredients to be absorbed through the skin.

Asian Mint Oil

Oil of an Asian mint, *Mentha arvensis* var. *piperascens,* is a constituent of many Chinese and Japanese oils and is especially rich in menthol. Menthol is anti-inflammatory, especially on the mucous membranes of the upper respiratory tract. It is also antimicrobial, a stimulant to mucosal secretions, and mildly anesthetic. For best results, use as an inhalation at the initial onset of symptoms.

Oils absorbed this way help ease infections and inflammations because they're often eliminated from the body through the lungs. One good technique is to apply the oil to the skin and then place a dry pack or towel on top to help the oils be absorbed and prevent evaporation. *Caution:* Thyme oil must be diluted in a base vegetable oil before being applied to the skin. People with high blood pressure should avoid this oil.

Recovery after Acute Bronchitis

After completing treatment, it's important to build on recovery by maintaining a healthy lifestyle: eating nutritious food, getting enough sleep and exercise, not smoking, and reducing stress. After acute bronchitis, a period of debility is common. The appropriate herbs will speed recovery and help the body recuperate. Respiratory tonics and bitter tonics should be emphasized, and so should herbs that support the particular body systems affected in each individual. Good tonics include coltsfoot, mullein, and horehound. Horehound, an excellent lung remedy with valuable bitter properties, is especially useful.

In the later stages of acute bronchitis, it's important to clear all the mucus from the lungs. Any of the expectorant essential oils used in inhalations, baths, and local massage to the chest and throat will help. These oils include the following:

- Basil
- Benzoin
- Bergamot
- Marjoram
- Myrrh
- Thyme
- Sandalwood

The cough may persist for a while after the fever has subsided, but using these oils will shorten the time to full recovery.

CHRONIC BRONCHITIS

Chronic bronchitis is defined as excessive mucus secretion in the bronchi and a chronic or recurrent mucus-producing cough that lasts for 3 or more months and recurs year after year. It is a long-term condition that does not involve fever.

Healthy lungs normally produce a small amount of mucus all the time. This mucus is continually swept out of the bronchi by the cilia. We don't notice this constant process because only a little mucus is produced, and it is swallowed imperceptibly with the saliva. In chronic bronchitis, which can be caused by infection, air pollution, smoking, or other external irritants, the body produces abnormally large amounts of mucus that literally swamp the cilia. Because the layer of mucus that covers the cilia is so thick, the cilia can no longer propel it upward. Coughing is the only way to expel the mucus.

Chronic bronchitis is often classified into three grades of severity. Simple chronic bronchitis is mild but persistent and is accompanied by clear sputum. In mucopurulent bronchitis, the sputum is occasionally or continually thick and is often yellowish because of bacterial infection. Obstructive bronchitis occurs when structural damage has been caused by continual infection, inflammation, and coughing. The bronchi become narrowed because the membrane that lines them thickens and scars. The lungs lose some of their elasticity, so breathing becomes more difficult. The amount of alveolar tissue — a very thin membrane through which oxygen enters the blood and through which waste material, such as carbon dioxide, is extracted — is reduced. Eventually, the heart may become overstrained because it repeatedly tries to maintain enough circulation in the lungs.

Chronic bronchitis may result from a series of attacks of acute bronchitis or may evolve gradually because of heavy smoking or inhalation of polluted air. When tobacco smoke is breathed into the lungs, it irritates the airways, which then produce mucus. Exposure for a long time to irritants such as fumes, dust, and other substances can generate chronic bronchitis. This condition is preventable since the primary causes are a range of pollutants. Climate and air pollution are serious factors in its development, but the two most important factors are smoking and poor nutrition.

Herbs to Consider for Chronic Bronchitis

When you're treating this chronic and debilitating condition, tonic support is vital. Herbal remedies are appropriate because they both address symptoms and strengthen the body as a whole. The respiratory, cardiovascular, and immune systems need attention. Some examples of useful tonics are:

- Pulmonary tonics, such as elecampane, which are essential for supporting the health and general tone of the lungs and the rest of the respiratory system
- Stimulating expectorants, like elecampane and horehound, which will help when there is excessive production of phlegm
- Relaxing expectorants, such as mullein, which may be helpful but are generally more effective in acute bronchitis
- Antispasmodics, like wild cherry bark, which may be helpful for severe coughing or breathlessness
- Antimicrobials, such as echinacea or garlic, which help the body eliminate any related bacterial infection of the lungs
- Cardiotonic herbs, such as hawthorn, which are essential for supporting cardiac function in the elderly or in people with weak hearts or longstanding chronic bronchitis

The Dietary Connection

Smokers are more likely to die of chronic bronchitis than of lung cancer. Giving up smoking is the first and most important preventive measure. The second is improving the nutrition in your diet. It's particularly important to cut out or greatly reduce intake of foods that encourage the production of mucus. For most people, that means dairy products and refined starches.

Of these two types of food, dairy products, including milk and cheese, seem to be the worst culprits. Restricting intake of these foods for several weeks or even several months will often produce an improvement. After such a period, cheese, milk, and other

---

Tea for Chronic Debilitating Bronchitis

This combination of stimulating and relaxing pulmonary tonics is formulated for a patient who is becoming debilitated and weakened by chronic bronchitis. Irish moss has long been used in Britain (the world's capital for chronic bronchitis!) as a nutritive support. Other herbs may be added to this to fit the needs of the individual, whether they be hawthorn, Siberian ginseng, or cleavers.

1 part elecampane	1 part coltsfoot
1 part irish moss	1 part mullein

To make: Combine the dried herbs and make an infusion using 1 teaspoon of the herb mixture for every 1 cup (240 ml) boiling water. Infuse for 20 minutes. See full instructions on page 113.

To use: Drink three times daily.

dairy foods may be cautiously reintroduced, but in very small amounts. Some people may have to omit them permanently. (Incidentally, goat's milk is found to be less mucus-forming than cow's milk.) Starches also provoke excessive mucus production, and refined starches (white flour and all products made from it) are much worse than unrefined grains. Additives, such as chemical flavorings, colorings, and preservatives, often trigger excess mucus production and should be avoided.

The best and simplest rule is to eat foods that are as near as possible to the condition in which they were grown. In other words, increase your intake of foods that haven't been processed, dried, frozen, packaged, or precooked. As often as possible, eat foods that are raw or have been cooked very slightly.

Tincture for Chronic Bronchitis Infection

This formula is intended for cases where the chronic bronchitis is associated with fever and an active infection.

1 part elecampane
1 part echinacea
1 part horehound
1 part mullein

To make: Combine dried or fresh herbs with alcohol to make a tincture, as instructed on page 115.
To make: Take 5 ml of the combination tincture three times a day. Supplement with a daily dose of garlic (raw or in capsule form).

Tincture for Chronic Bronchitis Congestion

This combination addresses a chronic bronchitis that is very productive and causes lung congestion.

1 part elecampane   1 part horehound
1 part bloodroot   1 part mullein

To make: Combine the dried or fresh herbs with alcohol to make a tincture, as instructed on page 115.
To use: Take 5 ml of the tincture combination three times daily. Supplement with a daily dose of garlic (raw or in capsule form).

Exercise for Chronic Bronchitis

Exercise can strengthen the muscles that help with breathing. It's important to try to exercise at least three times a week, at first gently and for just a little while. Slowly increase the duration and intensity of your exercise routine. For example, begin walking slowly for 15 minutes three times a week. Then, whenever you're feeling stronger, increase your walking speed and walk for a longer period — for example, walk for 20 to 25 minutes. Then increase the time to 30 minutes.

An exercise program called *pulmonary rehabilitation*, which is usually administered by a respiratory therapist, may help improve breathing. A method called *pursed-lip breathing* may also help. To perform pursed-lip breathing, take a deep breath and then breathe out slowly through the mouth while holding your lips as if you're preparing for a kiss. Pursed-lip breathing slows down the fast breathing that accompanies chronic bronchitis.

ASTHMA

Asthma is a chronic inflammatory disorder of the airways characterized by coughing, wheezing, chest tightness, and difficulty breathing. An estimated 15 million Americans suffer from asthma, including 4.8 million children and adolescents. Asthma can develop at any time but is most common in young children. When it starts in childhood, asthma usually improves with age. Adult-onset asthma often gets worse over time.

Many people think that asthma and wheezing are the same. This isn't true — wheezing is a sign of asthma, but it can also be caused by other things. Because of this confusion, the term *asthma* has been replaced with the more accurate term *reactive airway disease,* or RAD.

Symptoms

In people with asthma, the bronchial passages are very sensitive to irritation. This hypersensitivity inflames the tiny airways deep in the lungs. Consequently, excess mucus is produced and the muscles that wind around the bronchial tubes tighten. The combination of swelling, mucus, and muscle tightening narrows the airways. Wheezing (whistling and labored breathing) usually results, but a dry cough is sometimes the only sign.

Because the passages are narrowed and air flow reduced, mucus also builds up in the lungs, and this makes it even more difficult to breathe. The mucus is also a breeding ground for bacteria, so attacks of bronchitis may arise as a complication of the asthma. The following are classic symptoms of asthma:

- Wheezing. A low or loud whistle, usually heard during exhalation
- Coughing. A persistent mild cough or hack that often occurs at night
- Chest tightness. A burning sensation or a feeling of bands being strapped around the chest

• Shortness of breath. A feeling of trying to breathe through a straw (exhaling is especially difficult)

These symptoms usually occur when someone is exposed to certain "triggers" that initiate an attack. When an attack begins, a sequence of events occurs in the lungs. Here's what happens:

• Swelling. The bronchial tubes, often already swollen because of chronic asthma, become even more inflamed; this reduces the amount of air that can move in and out of the lungs.
• Tightening. The muscles around the tubes squeeze together (a process called *bronchoconstriction*), making breathing difficult.
• Clogging. The tubes start to make more mucus, which clogs the airways.

Asthma Triggers

Many asthma attacks are triggered by allergens, such as dust, mold spores, mites, animal hair, or feathers, but the onset may equally be caused by cold air or may be preceded by an infection such as a cold. Certainly, stress and, more specifically, acute anxiety are known to be the immediate triggers for many attacks, and this can sometimes give rise to a vicious circle of asthma — anxiety about the asthma leads to further attacks. Thus a wide range of etiological factors can be involved in this all-too-common problem.

Asthma can be classified into two general groupings defined by the trigger:

> ## Foods That May Trigger Asthma
>
> Ingested allergens can be a trigger for asthma. These could include foods, medications (such as aspirin, colored pills, capsules, or syrups), food additives, yeasts, and molds.

• **Extrinsic asthma** is caused by allergic responses to house dust, animal fur, or various foods. Such causes account for 10 to 20 percent of adult asthma cases.

WHEN TO SEEK IMMEDIATE MEDICAL ATTENTION

Asthma can be an extremely serious condition. Herbal medicine has much to offer in the treatment, control, and even cure of asthmatic problems, but it will not replace emergency medical support if indicated. You should see a doctor immediately if:

- You experience shortness of breath or rapid breathing even when resting.
- You experience chest wall retraction—in other words, the muscles between your ribs suck inward with each breath. This means that too much force is required to suck air into the bronchial tubes, and you should seek treatment to widen the airways immediately.
- Your sleep is disturbed by coughing or wheezing.
- You become much more dependent on inhalers. If you find yourself using your inhaler more often than your doctor has recommended, or if your average use has increased by more than 50 percent, you may need to adjust your treatment program.

- **Intrinsic asthma** is caused by genetics, structural problems, infections, pollutants, and stress (both physiological and psychological). Such causes account for 30 to 50 percent of adult asthma cases.

Allergies. An estimated 75 percent of childhood asthma is allergy related. Controlling allergies is pivotal to reducing the frequency of asthma attacks. If asthma symptoms worsen during certain seasons, it's probably because of plant pollen. When exposed to pollen, the body may respond by creating antibodies that attach themselves to special cells, called *mast cells*, in the nose and airways. The mast cells produce and release a chemical called *histamine*. Histamine causes allergy symptoms.

Tree pollens trigger problems in early spring, grass pollens strike in late spring and early summer, and weed pollens cause flare-ups in late summer. Allergy seasons begin at different times in different places. For example, on the East Coast and in the

Midwest, ragweed strikes hardest from mid-August to late October. It's very important to learn your area's seasonal patterns.

Gastric reflux (heartburn). Reflux problems may cause up to 30 percent of all cases of asthma. Even when other triggers for asthma have been identified, preventing heartburn can make a difference. Heartburn often occurs at night because it's easier for stomach acid to seep into the esophagus or throat when people are lying down. If acid leaks into the breathing passages, it can cause choking and wheezing.

Colds and other respiratory infections. These are the most common asthma triggers. In asthmatic people, even mild head colds can inflame the airways very quickly.

Air pollution. Cigarette and wood smoke, chemical vapors, irritating gases, perfumes, and dust can all be problems for people with asthma.

Weather. Cold, dry air is more aggravating to asthma than warm, moist air. Simple measures, like breathing through a scarf or taking preventive medicines before exercising on cold days, will help minimize attacks. Weather changes, such as shifts in barometric pressure, humidity, or temperature, can also trigger attacks.

Childhood–Onset Asthma

Asthma that begins in childhood is closely linked to the presence of eczema, hay fever, urticaria, and migraines in the patient or in close relatives. People with a family history of these disorders are considered to be atopic. If both parents have a history of atopy, their child has a 75 percent chance of being affected; if only one parent is affected, there's a 50 percent chance that the child will be, too. In comparison, if neither parent is affected, the chance that the child will develop asthma is 12 percent. Episodic coughing often precedes childhood asthma for several months or even years, later developing into wheezy bronchitis and then asthma. Children who develop asthma often have a prior history of slow recovery from upper respiratory infections.

Adult-Onset Asthma

Adult-onset asthma is more common in women than in men. There are two main types of adult-onset asthma. In the first type, asthma attacks seem to happen randomly, for no obvious reason. In the second, there are usually fairly obvious "triggers." After the triggers are determined, the sufferer can try to avoid them, but even so, new triggers may develop.

Herbs to Consider for Asthma

Many herbs can help relieve asthma. For example:

- Expectorants are essential in reducing the buildup of mucus in the lungs. However, stimulant expectorants may aggravate breathing difficulties. It's best to use only relaxing expectorants, such as mullein.
- Antispasmodics, like lobelia, help relieve the spasm response in the muscles of the lungs.
- Antimicrobial herbs, such as echinacea or garlic, are indicated when there's a danger of secondary infections, which must be prevented at all costs.
- Cardiotonic herbs, such as hawthorn or motherwort, support the heart when the lungs are congested.
- Nervine herbs, such as skullcap or chamomile, are helpful because stress is always a factor in asthma, either as a trigger or as a result.
- Ma huang can be very useful as a bronchodilator. It contains the alkaloid ephedrine, which helps relieve the bronchial spasms that underlie asthma attacks. Ma huang is also helpful for treating allergic reactions because it acts on the sympathetic nerves. Other plants from around the world have marked antispasmodic and bronchodilating effects. The most important ones within Western herbalism are grindelia, sundew, and wild cherry bark.

Tincture for Asthma

This formula incorporates the herbs most commonly cited in Western herbalism for their effectiveness in easing muscle tension and opening up the bronchial passages.

4 parts grindelia
1 part lobelia
1 part wild cherry bark

1 part licorice
1 part motherwort
1 part ma huang

To make: Combine all herbs in alcohol to make a tincture (see page 115 for full instructions.)
To use: Take 5 ml of the tincture combination three times a day.

Tincture for Atopic Asthma in Children

This formula is specially designed to address the needs of children with a family history of asthma.

1 part Cleavers
1 part Red clover
1 part Nettle leaf

2 parts Tincture for Asthma
(see recipe above)

To make: Combine the cleavers, red clover, and nettle leaf with alcohol to make a tincture (see page 115 for full instructions). Add Tincture for Asthma and shake well.
To use: Take 5 ml of the tincture combination three times a day.

Addressing Related Emotional Factors

It's obvious that our lungs are connected to our emotions — think of how your lungs feel when you're laughing or crying. Because people with asthma have impaired lung function, they may find it physically impossible to express their emotions. It's worth exploring the possible emotional or psychological issues that may be contributing to the physical symptoms. This could be done through self-reflection or professional counseling.

Other alternative health practices, such as deep breathing (as taught in practices such as yoga), can strengthen our connection to our feelings. Breathing exercises will help alleviate asthma when practiced regularly. Exercise in general, such as walking, swimming, yoga, tai chi, and relaxation, will also help deepen and relax breathing.

Bach flower remedies are also helpful in addressing emotional issues that may be aggravating the asthma. This is a unique healing system developed by Dr. Edward Bach that consists of essences made from 38 different flowers. Just as the body has its own self-healing properties regarding physical diseases and symptoms, the mind and spirit have their own self-healing capacities, which the Bach flower remedies stimulate. The remedies are prepared from the flowers of wild plants, bushes, and trees, and none of them is harmful or habitforming.

Each flower remedy is used to address a particular state of mind or mood, such as worry, apprehension, hopelessness, or irritability. These long-term worries or fears are important to address because they can deplete an individual's vitality. Emotional states may hinder recovery of health, retard convalescence, or even contribute to sickness and disease.

In selecting a particular Bach flower remedy, you must first identify the individual's unique mental pattern, based on attitude, feelings, worries, and the degree to which the person is plagued by qualities such as indecision, timidity, resentment, vexations, possessiveness, hopelessness, lethargy, hatred, an overpowering or demanding nature, intolerance, or tension. Most important, to select the correct remedy, you need to determine why there is apprehension, worry, and fear. For a complete list of the remedies and their application, see the chart below.

Since the Bach flower remedies are benign in their action and can result in no unpleasant reactions, they can be taken by anyone. Stick concentrate remedies will keep indefinitely. A 10 ml concentrate bottle will make approximately 60 treatments.

A GUIDE TO BACH FLOWER REMEDIES

REMEDY	APPLICATION
Agrimony	Suffering from torture that is hidden behind a facade of cheerfulness. Often used as a remedy for alcoholism.
Aspen	Apprehensive — feeling that something dreadful is going to happen without knowing why. Unexplainable fear, anxiety, and presentiments.
Beech	Critical and intolerant of others. Arrogant.
Centaury	Weak willed. Those who let themselves be exploited or imposed upon, become subservient, and have difficulty saying "no."
Cerato	Doubting personal judgment or intuition; seeking advice of others. Often influenced and misguided.
Cherry plum	Subject to uncontrolled, irrational thoughts. Fear of losing control and doing something terrible; fear of "going crazy." Uncontrolled bursts of temper. Impulsive suicide.
Chestnut bud	Refusing to learn by experience; continually repeating the same mistakes.
Chicory	Overly possessive; demands respect or attention; likes others to conform to his or her standards. Makes martyr of oneself. Interferes and manipulates.
Clematis	Indifferent, inattentive, daydreaming, absentminded. Mental escapist from reality.
Crab apple	Feels unclean or ashamed of ailments. Self-disgust or hatred. House proud. (Crab apple is known as "the cleanser flower.")

Remedies can also be combined — 2 drops of each chosen remedy in a glass of water — and sipped at intervals, or mixed in a 30 ml (1 ounce) dropper bottle filled with spring water from which 4 drops are directly placed on the tongue at least 4 times a day. If the mixture tends to spoil or get sour, which may happen (especially in warm weather), you can add whisky, gin, or cognac in a 20 percent ratio as a preservative. If you want to avoid alcohol, use 50 percent cider vinegar or rice vinegar instead.

REMEDY	APPLICATION
Elm	Temporarily overcome by inadequacy or responsibility, though normally very capable.
Gentian	Despondent. Easily discouraged and rejected. Skeptical, pessimistic. Depression, where the cause is known.
Gorse	Desperate, without hope. "Oh, what's the use." Defeatism.
Heather	Obsessed with personal troubles and experiences. Talkative bores, poor listeners.
Holly	Jealous, envious, revengeful, and suspicious. Those who hate.
Honeysuckle	Nostalgic and constantly dwelling in the past. Homesickness.
Hornbeam	"Monday morning" feeling, but once started, task is usually fulfilled. Mentally tired. Procrastination.
Impatiens	Impatience, irritability. Reacts in an exaggerated manner.
Larch	Despondency due to lack of self-confidence. Expectation of failure, so fails to make any attempt. Feels inferior, yet has the ability.
Mimulus	Fear of known things; fear of the world. Shyness, timidity, bashfulness.
Mustard	"Dark cloud" of depression that descends for no known reason and can lift just as suddenly, making one downcast, saddened, and low.
Oak	Brave, determined. Struggles on in illness and against adversity despite setbacks. Plodders, never resting.
Olive	Drained of energy; everything is an effort. Physically fatigued.
Pine	Feeling guilty. Blames oneself for the mistakes of others. Feels unworthy.

A GUIDE TO BACH FLOWER REMEDIES — continued

REMEDY	APPLICATION
Red chestnut	Excessive care of and concern for others, especially those held dear.
Rescue Remedy	Includes five specific remedies (cherry, clematis, plum, rock rose, star of Bethlehem) formulated for emergency use. Purpose is to comfort, reassure, and calm those who have received serious news, severe upset, or startling experiences and have consequently fallen into a numbed, bemused state of mind. Rescue Remedy is invaluable to keep at hand for immediate use. It does not take the place of medical attention. It is taken orally (4 drops in a glass of water) but can also be applied externally either in a liquid or cream form.
Rock rose	Alarmed, panicky, full of trepidation.
Rock water	Hard on oneself, often overworked. Rigid-minded, self-denying. Ascetic.
Scleranthus	Uncertainty, indecision, vacillation. Fluctuating moods.
Star of Bethlehem	All effects of serious news or fright following an accident. Release from trauma, no matter how old it is.
Sweet chestnut	Absolute dejection. Feels at the limit of what one can stand.
Vervain	Overenthusiasm, overeffort, straining. Fanatical and high strung. Incensed and frustrated by injustices.

Dietary Changes

Try to identify food sensitivities that may be contributing to asthma. Some people may find that it helps to temporarily avoid eggs, wheat, gluten (found in wheat, oats, barley, and rye), and dairy products. Other questionable items are alcohol and preserved fruit, which often contains sulfur dioxide. Many people with asthma have a negative reaction to foods with amounts of sulfur dioxide as small as five parts per million.

It may also be helpful to use the following nutritional supplements: vitamin B_6 (25 mg twice daily), vitamin B_{12} (100 mcg daily), vitamin C (1,000 to 2,000 mg daily), vitamin E (400 IU

REMEDY	APPLICATION
Vine	Dominating, inflexible, ambitious, tyrannical, autocratic. Arrogant pride. Good leadership.
Walnut	Protects against powerful influences and helps adjustment to any transition or change (e.g., puberty, menopause, divorce, new surroundings). Contrary to those who benefit from centaury (see page 54), the person knows what he wants but is easily influenced by other people to do something else.
Water violet	Proud, reserved, sedate, sometimes "superior." Little emotional involvement, but reliable and dependable.
White chestnut	Persistent unwanted thoughts. Preoccupation with some worry or episode. Mental arguments. Constant inner dialogue.
Wild oat	Helps determine one's intended path of life.
Wild rose	Resignation, apathy. Drifters who accept their lot, making little or no effort for improvement. Lack of ambition.
Willow	Resentment and bitterness with "not fair" and "poor me" attitude.

daily), and selenium (250 mcg daily), as suggested by Drs. Pizzorno and Murray in *The Textbook of Natural Medicine.*

Massage and Aromatherapy

The whole thoracic area, both the back and the chest, should be massaged on a regular basis, with particular emphasis on strokes that "open out" the chest and shoulders. The use of essential oils depends on many factors, such as whether infection is present, whether the asthma is known to be an allergic response, and whether emotional factors have triggered the attack.

During an actual crisis, inhalation of an antispasmodic oil is the only practical herbal remedy. Sniffing directly from the bottle of oil or smelling some drops on a tissue is safer than inhaling steam; this is because the heat from the steam will increase any inflammation of the mucous membranes and worsen the congestion.

Essential oils that are useful for inhalation include:

- Hyssop
- Aniseed
- Lavender
- Pine
- Rosemary

MAINTAINING UPPER RESPIRATORY SYSTEM HEALTH

As with many modern health problems, prevention of ailments of the upper respiratory system is largely a matter of avoiding pollutants and watching your diet. Air pollution will aggravate or even cause a whole spectrum of problems. This includes both particulate matter and irritant gases, so stop smoking and move out of Los Angeles! Many of the common chronic respiratory or catarrhal ailments are a response by the body to a diet that is too rich in mucus-forming foods. So, for someone with such problems, a low-mucous diet is essential.

Patterns of Disease

There are some basic patterns of disease that affect the upper respiratory system. By understanding the phytotherapy (or herbal medicine) approach to each, treatments for diverse pathologies become surprisingly straightforward. Four basic factors must always be taken into consideration in any evaluation of a respiratory condition. These include:

Allergic response. The allergen must be identified and, if possible, removed from the affected person's environment. This may be easy to do if the trigger is a food sensitivity but is much more problematic if the trigger is a ubiquitous environmental factor, such as pollen or house dust. The approach to discerning allergens is discussed in the section on hayfever (see page 68).

Congestion. Blockage of the sinus cavities with catarrh (mucus) is very common and is relatively easy to treat with herbs. However, it is not always appropriate to "dry up" such overproduction of the normal secretions. If the body is using the mucous membranes of the sinuses as a window for removing waste within the vehicle of the catarrh, then it is best to support this rather than block it. This is discussed in more depth in the sections that follow. The production of excessive and thick mucus in the nose and other respiratory passages is a response to any inflammation of the mucus membrane that lines them. Inflammation can be caused by an infection, autoimmune problems, or irritants such as pollutants, pollens, and dust.

Infection. Acute infections of the nose, sinuses, and throat are all too common! Occasional acute infections are treated in a straightforward way with antimicrobials, essential oils, and anticatarrhals. However, if there is a recurrent pattern of frequent infection, attention must be given to the whole body, and a treatment focused on supporting the immune system should be given.

Physical blockage. Any sign of obstruction in the passages calls for skilled diagnostic investigations. Some benign problems, such as nasal polyps, are treatable with herbs, but differential diagnosis is vital.

Anticatarrhal

Catarrh is defined as an inflammation of a mucous membrane with an associated increase of mucus, especially affecting the nose and throat. Mucus is a thin, slippery, protective fluid secreted by mucous membranes and glands; it becomes thick and sticky in a number of diseases.

The anticatarrhal herbs help the body to remove excess mucus buildups, whether in the sinus area or other parts of the body.

Mucus and catarrh are not in themselves a problem. Mucus is an essential body product, but when too much is produced it is often in response to an infection, or as a way of helping the body remove the problematic organism or excess carbohydrates from the body. In such cases a low–mucus-forming diet is called for.

Some of these remedies work by producing a more watery mucus secretion, enabling the body to remove it; others reduce the secretion directly. This is not as desirable as it sounds, as it may cause a buildup of waste that cannot be cleared from the sinuses.

Tonics for the Upper Respiratory System

Nature is abundant in herbs that have an anticatarrhal effect upon the upper respiratory system, but this is not the same as being a tonic for that part of the body. Simply affecting tissue or function does not equate automatically with the nurturing quality of a tonic. However, defining adequately what a tonic is has proven too challenging for this author! Suffice it to say that tonics are plants that in some way increase the vitality of a tissue, organ, or body system. From the European perspective, the herb list for addressing the needs of this system includes goldenseal, goldenrod, elder, eyebright, and hyssop.

Anticatarrhal Herbs

Bearberry	Elecampane	Irish moss	Yarrow
Boneset	Eyebright	Marsh mallow	
Cayenne	Garlic	Mullein	
Coltsfoot	Goldenrod	Peppermint	
Cranesbill	Goldenseal	Sage	
Echinacea	Hyssop	Thyme	
Elder	Iceland moss	Wild indigo	

COMMON COLD

The common cold, a viral infection of the upper respiratory tract, is one of the banes of life. Many different, constantly mutating strains of viruses cause cold symptoms. Most colds aren't serious. However, the mucous membranes of the nose and throat are much more vulnerable to attack by bacteria when they become inflamed from the infection. This vulnerability makes it easier for secondary infections, such as sinusitis, ear infections, and bronchitis, to develop. Antibiotic drugs, which destroy bacteria, can't harm a cold virus. Because viral infections can't be cured, a doctor can't do more for you than you can do for yourself.

There is no universally miraculous herbal cold cure! However, herbal medicine can do more than most therapies in treating and preventing this all-too-common problem. By selecting herbs that fit the individual's unique needs and addressing issues such as immune support, diet, and lifestyle, we are able to take on the common cold without a problem.

Prevention

Traditional remedies can ease the aches, pains, and general discomfort caused by viral infections. If you frequently get colds, your body is hinting that your immune system needs help. Echinacea, goldenseal, and garlic can increase the vitality of your immune response.

Foot Bath for the Common Cold

A foot bath is a traditional treatment for cold symptoms. Dissolve 1 tablespoon of mustard powder in 4 pints (2 L) of hot water. Bathe the feet for 10 minutes, twice a day.

Treating Symptoms

When you get a cold, you need to address your symptoms and support your body's fight against the virus. Aches and pains are common, and many herbs will relieve them. The best remedy may be the diaphoretic boneset, especially when fever is involved. Chamomile, linden flower, and peppermint tea may have similar effects. Although they aren't as strong as boneset, they taste much better. Boneset's bitter taste produces one of its therapeutic qualities, but most people don't enjoy it.

Congestion is the body's normal response to infection, so don't try to relieve it with anticatarrhal drugs. Herbal anticatarrhals are safer than nonherbal ones because they work in a different way. Chamomile, peppermint, and boneset will relieve a lot of the discomfort. Goldenseal, raw garlic, and garlic oil capsules will speed healing, and steam inhalations of eucalyptus and thyme oils will reduce catarrh formation.

To help the immune system, use antimicrobial herbs, such as echinacea and goldenseal, and the tonics cleavers or nettles. These may be combined in capsules or used as tinctures.

Herbs to Consider for the Common Cold

- Antimicrobials, such as echinacea, will help the immune system combat the viral infection and prevent secondary infections.
- Anticatarrhals, such as elderflower, ease the symptomatic discomfort that's characteristic of the common cold. However, as discussed, you don't want to "dry up" the overproduction of mucus by using decongestants.
- Diaphoretics, such as yarrow, help relieve fever and support the body as it copes with elevated temperature.
- Expectorants are called for when secondary problems develop in the lower respiratory system.

For short-term infections, systemic support is usually unnecessary. However, if you get recurrent colds, tonic remedies are vital. Immune support is important, and so is dealing with the stress in your life. If your colds tend to develop into coughs or bronchitis, pulmonaries are called for. If you have a history of heart disease, it may be important to use cardiac tonics (such as linden) as a precaution. In this case, linden would be most appropriate, as it is also a diaphoretic, although it does not replace hawthorn.

Steam Inhalation for Colds

Several essential oil treatments will help diminish the discomfort of a cold and reduce the risk for secondary infections. For the immediate relief of congestion and to soothe inflamed mucous membranes, a steam inhalation using essential oils is often effective. The antiviral effects of oils such as eucalyptus and tea tree will also help inhibit the virus. Very hot steam — as hot as you can tolerate without burning your nose and throat — creates an environment that's hostile to viruses. The addition of an antiviral oil increases the effectiveness of the steam. Lavender, peppermint, rosemary, eucalyptus, thyme, and tea tree are all good oils to use. They ease congestion and also help combat infection.

A steam inhalation with appropriate essential oils has several beneficial effects. It clears the congested nasal passages and soothes the inflamed mucous membrane. At the same time, the essential oils kill many bacteria. Some of the oils, especially eucalyptus and tea tree, inhibit the cold virus. You can also use fresh herbs, as when making a steam inhalation.

To make a steam inhalation, place the essential oils or fresh herbs in a large bowl and pour in boiling water. Drape a towel over your head to create a "tent." Lean over the bowl and trap the steam, breathing deeply. A good combination for treating colds is equal parts chamomile flowers, thyme, and marjoram used in the proportion of 1 tablespoon of the herb mixture to .5 L (1.7 ounces) boiling water.

Herbs for Treating Colds

Diaphoretics
Cayenne
Elder
Garlic
Horseradish
Linden
Mustard
Onion
Peppermint
Yarrow

Antimicrobials
Echinacea
Eucalyptus
Garlic
Onion
Thyme

Elder-Peppermint-Yarrow Infusion for Colds

This classic northern European combination has been valued for generations as a treatment for the unpleasant symptoms of a cold.

1 part elder
1 part yarrow
1 part peppermint

To make: Combine all ingredients. Add 1–2 teaspoons of the herb mixture to 1 cup (240 ml) boiling water and infuse for 20 minutes. See page 113 for full instructions.

To use: Drink the hot tea as often as needed until the symptoms pass.

Spice Drink

Many traditional cold remedies use culinary ingredients, highlighting the fact that medicinal and culinary plants both have healing properties. At the first sign of a chill or sore throat, try the following hot drink made from common kitchen spices.

1 cinnamon stick, broken into pieces
3 cloves
1 teaspoon coriander seeds
1 ounce (30 g) ginger, freshly sliced
1 lemon slice
1 pint (500 ml) water

To make: Combine all the ingredients in a saucepan. Make a decoction by cooking for 15 minutes, as directed on page 114. Strain. Sweeten to taste with organic honey.

To use: Drink the hot liquid every 2 hours.

If you are using essential oils, you might want to use a combination of eucalyptus and tea tree (or, as an alternative, rosemary and peppermint) early in the day, as these oils are mildly stimulating. At night, try an inhalation of lavender or a bath with a few drops of lavender oil added. You might also want to use lavender oils in an aromatherapy diffuser in your bedroom at night, especially if you are suffering from a cough.

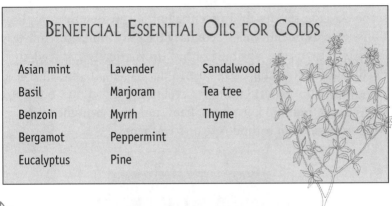

BENEFICIAL ESSENTIAL OILS FOR COLDS

Asian mint	Lavender	Sandalwood
Basil	Marjoram	Tea tree
Benzoin	Myrrh	Thyme
Bergamot	Peppermint	
Eucalyptus	Pine	

FLU

Influenza, commonly called the flu, is a severe viral respiratory tract infection that has generalized bodily symptoms. New mutations of the virus arise all the time, which is why immunity against one strain (resulting from previous exposure or immunization) does not protect against other strains. New types of flu spread very quickly, causing serious illness and many deaths.

Consider the mortality rates associated with some flu pandemics over the past 100 years:

- 1918–1919: The Spanish flu caused the highest known rate of flu-related mortality. There were approximately 500,000 deaths in the United States and 20 million worldwide.
- 1957–1958: The Asian flu killed 70,000 people in the United States.
- 1968–1969: The Hong Kong flu was responsible for 34,000 deaths in the United States.

Symptoms of flu include high fever (temperatures of 100°F to 103°F in adults and even higher in children), cough, sore throat, runny or stuffy nose, headache, muscle aches, and often extreme fatigue. There may be nausea, vomiting, and diarrhea, although gastrointestinal symptoms aren't usually prominent. The term *stomach flu* is a misnomer because gastrointestinal illnesses aren't usually caused by flu viruses.

Most people recover completely from flu in 1 to 2 weeks, but some develop serious and potentially life-threatening complications, such as pneumonia. Secondary bacterial infections are very serious. The use of antibiotics has dramatically reduced such deaths, although young children and elderly people are still at risk. It's sensible to use antibiotics for secondary infections, but don't discontinue herbal treatments. They can only be beneficial and won't conflict with orthodox drug treatment.

Goldenseal-Echinacea Flu Remedy

This tincture formula combines two strong immune-system boosters.

1 part goldenseal
1 part echinacea

To make: Combine herbs with alcohol to make a tincture as directed on page 115.
To use: Take 2.5 ml of the tincture every 2 hours. Supplement with a strong infusion of boneset, drunk hot once every hour.

Herbs to Consider for Flu

- Antimicrobials, such as goldenseal and echinacea, help the immune system combat the viral infection and prevent secondary infections.
- Diaphoretics, such as boneset, help relieve fever and support the body as it copes with the elevated temperature.
- Anticatarrhals, such as elderflower, ease the symptomatic discomfort characteristic of the flu.
- Expectorants are called for when secondary problems cause mucus buildup in the lower respiratory system.
- Bitters, mainly boneset, help relieve the debility that often occurs with viral infections.

Unfortunately, the flu is another condition that has no miracle cure. However, herbal medicines will go a long way toward making life much more bearable while the infection lasts.

Other Treatment Options

Treatments for flu are most effective when they are started at the first sign of infection. Taking a moderately hot bath and adding a few drops of antiviral essential oil — for example, tea tree — to the water will often induce diaphoresis and then a deep, restful sleep. (Keep in mind, however, that tea tree sometimes mildly irritates the skin. Some people may not be able to tolerate more than three or four drops in a full bath.) This treatment may be enough to avert a full-blown attack, but it's a good idea to repeat it several times over the next 2 or 3 days.

When to Seek Medical Attention

You should see a doctor if you experience such symptoms as cloudy consciousness or breathlessness. You should also see a doctor if symptoms continue steadily for more than 1 week, or if you seem to be recovering and then suddenly get worse. Secondary infections, like chest infections and pneumonia, are common when the body's defenses are down.

People often recover slowly from the flu. Stimulant herbs that contain caffeine should be avoided because they provide only a temporary "lift" and the caffeine may delay full recovery. Bitter tonics speed recovery through their metabolic-stimulating effects. Appropriate bitter tonics include:

- **Boneset,** which is also diaphoretic and anticatarrhal
- **Gentian,** which aids digestion and has a tolerable taste
- **Goldenseal,** which is also anticatarrhal and generally tonic
- **White horehound,** which is an expectorant and anticatarrhal

It may be helpful to take a multivitamin and mineral supplement until your appetite and general vitality are back to normal.

Hay Fever

Hay fever is an allergy that affects the lining of the nose and, often, the eyes and throat. As the name implies, it's an allergic response to the pollen of certain grasses. It may also occur in reaction to the spores of some fungi. Hay fever responds well to herbal medicine, although every person reacts differently. You may have to try various approaches until you find the right one.

Ma huang *(Ephedra sinica)* is the only herb specifically indicated for hay fever. You should consult a comprehensive herbal guide or an herbal practitioner before using it. Apart from using ma huang, the most effective approach is to address symptoms.

Herbs to Consider for Hay Fever

- Anticatarrhals, such as goldenseal, chamomile, goldenrod, and boneset, will ease the symptomatic discomfort that often characterizes hay fever. However, don't try to "dry up" the overproduction of mucus. This can be very uncomfortable.
- Expectorants are needed when wheezing or pulmonary congestion is present. Consider relaxing expectorants, such as mullein.

- Bitters help tone the body so that it can better deal with the immune system's response.
- For dry and irritated eyes, use a wash of chamomile applied directly on the eyes or apply a thin slice of fresh cucumber to your closed eyelids.
- Nettles can be used to help ease the body's underlying sensitivity to allergens.

Essential Oils for Hay Fever

Many essential oils will help ease hay fever symptoms. You can add the oils to hot water for a steam inhalation or put some oil on a tissue and sniff as needed. Helpful oils include blue chamomile, lemon balm, and lavender. You may also want to use these oils as a massage application.

Hay Fever Tincture

For greatest effectiveness, start this treatment 2 months before hay fever season begins.

1 part ma huang	2 parts nettles
1 part goldenseal	2 parts goldenrod
1 part eyebright	

To make: Combine herbs with alcohol to make a tincture, as described on page 115.

To use: Take 5 ml of the combination tincture three times daily. If you start 2 months in advance of hay fever season, as suggested, increase the dosage gradually, according to the following schedule (for adults only):

Weeks 1 to 2 — 2.5 ml once daily
Weeks 3 to 4 — 5 ml once daily
Weeks 5 to 6 — 5 ml twice daily
Weeks 7 to 8 — 5 ml three times daily

SINUSITIS

The sinuses are air spaces in the bones around the nose and eyes. They reduce the weight of the skull and also act as resonators — they're responsible for creating the unique sound of each person's voice.

The tissue that lines the sinuses produces mucus. The sinuses help warm and moisturize incoming air. Microscopic hair cells in the sinuses, called cilia, continually sweep out mucus and move it into the nose. Anything that blocks the tiny sinus openings or impedes the cilia can cause a sinus infection or inflammation of the mucous membranes. This occurs because the buildup of mucus creates an ideal environment for microorganisms to thrive in. Sinusitis is usually caused by upper respiratory infections, hay fever or other allergies, cigarette smoke, air pollution, air travel, or swimming under water.

Herbs for Sinusitis

- Antimicrobials are pivotal in the treatment of this often stubborn condition. These herbs help the body deal with any infection, and they support the immune system in resisting possible secondary infections. Examples include echinacea and wild indigo.
- Anticatarrhals, such as elderflower and goldenrod, ease the symptomatic discomfort characteristic of sinusitis and also help the body remove mucus buildups in the sinus cavities.
- Astringents, which are often anticatarrhals, such as elder-flower and yarrow, reduce the amount of mucus produced by the sinus membranes.
- Anti-inflammatories are indicated, but most of the other herbs used to treat sinusitis also have this effect.
- Diaphoretics, such as yarrow and elderflower, may be needed to reduce fever if it occurs.

Tincture for Sinusitis

This formula includes herbs with antimicrobial, anticatarrhal, and astringent properties.

2 parts goldenrod	1 part echinacea
1 part elderflower	1 part wild indigo

To make: Combine herbs with alcohol to make a tincture, as directed on page 115.
To use: Take 5 ml of the tincture three times daily.

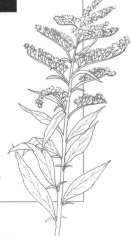

Treatment Approach

Sometimes overproduction of mucus is the body's attempt to discharge waste material that is not being properly eliminated by the bowels, kidneys, and skin. In such cases, herbalists may recommend bitter tonics to encourage regular bowel movements. Diuretic herbs can be used to encourage the kidneys to eliminate retained fluids. The diaphoretic herbs help stimulate elimination through the skin.

It's important to establish a diet that reduces mucus production. In particular, a 2- or 3-day fruit-only fast will help clear a system clogged and overburdened by harmful wastes. You can also reduce mucus production with hot lemon drinks, garlic, onions, and horseradish. You can grate fresh horseradish root into cider vinegar or lemon juice and have a little each day. You can also add mustard and aromatic herbs, such as oregano, to your food. Taking zinc and vitamin C supplements will help increase the body's resistance to infection.

Certain foods can help alleviate sinusitis; others may contribute to it. Wheat and dairy foods, which promote the excessive formation of mucus, seem to predispose many people toward sinusitis. During an acute attack of sinusitis, it's helpful to avoid all dairy- and wheat-based foods for several days. People who have frequent attacks of sinusitis may need to give up these foods completely for several months and then reintroduce them in very small amounts, if at all. Goat's and sheep's milk may be better tolerated than cow's milk.

Sometimes emotional factors can result in respiratory problems. For example, suppressed grief can lead to blocked upper respiratory passages. A good cry will help free this blocked energy and alleviate the problem.

Steam Treatment for Sinusitis

This essential oil combination offers a strong inhalation for immediate soothing relief.

- 30 ml compound tincture of benzoin
- 2.5 ml eucalyptus essential oil
- 6 drops peppermint essential oil
- 5 drops lavender essential oil
- 5 drops pine essential oil
- 1 pint (500 ml) boiling water

To make: Combine all ingredients except water in a bottle and shake well.

To use: Put 1 teaspoon of the mixture in a bowl and add the boiling water. Drape a towel around your head to trap the steam, lean over the bowl, and breathe deeply. The vapor may be irritating, so keep your eyes closed.

SORE THROAT

A sore throat is often the first symptom of a cold or the flu. The usual cause of a sore throat is a viral infection, although bacterial infections can cause it, too. A sore throat is often accompanied by enlarged, tender glands in the neck. This is no cause for concern; it just means that the body's defense mechanisms are battling the infection. However, if neck stiffness is associated with the swollen glands, you should ask your doctor to rule out meningitis. You should also call your doctor when a sore throat persists for more than 1 week.

LARYNGITIS

Laryngitis is an acute inflammation of the larynx, or voice box. It's usually associated with a common cold or overuse of the voice and is characterized by swelling, hoarseness, pain, throat dryness, coughing, and an inability to speak above a whisper, if at all. Most laryngitis is caused by bacterial or viral infection. The infection may be restricted to the larynx or may be part of a more general infection of the upper respiratory tract.

Many herbs can be used for conditions that affect the mouth, larynx, and pharynx. Osha can be very helpful. Chewing a small piece of the root will help relieve symptoms and will promote the body's immune response. In Europe, the traditional approach to laryngitis has been to gargle with astringent herbs. (The liquids should not be swallowed because they can cause constipation, an unnecessary and unfortunate complication.) Helpful astringent herbs for laryngitis include:

- Blackberry leaves
- Cranesbill
- Elderflower
- Oak bark
- Raspberry leaves
- Sage
- Yarrow

Dietary Advice

To learn what dietary changes may help relieve the symptoms of laryngitis, see the supplement and dietary advice given for sinusitis on page 71. These guidelines apply to laryngitis, as well.

Laryngitis Tincture

This formula includes strong herbs for supporting the immune system.

- 2 parts echinacea
- 2 parts osha
- 1 part goldenseal

To make: Combine herbs with alcohol to make a tincture, as described on page 115.
To use: Take 1 ml of the tincture every hour.

Gargle for Laryngitis

This formula helps ease inflammation and irritation in the throat.

- 1 part sage
- 1 part chamomile

To make: Combine herbs in a bowl or teapot and cover with boiling water to make a strong infusion, as directed on page 113. Allow to cool before use.
To use: Gargle often until symptoms subside.

> ## An Alternate Gargle for Laryngitis
>
> *Be sure to use the essential oils in this recipe in the limited quantity directed.*
>
> 3 drops oil of cypress or oil of bergamot
> ½ cup (120 ml) warm water
>
> **To make:** Put the oil of cypress or oil of bergamot drops in the warm water.
> **To use:** Gargle every hour to reduce inflammation.

TONSILLITIS

Tonsillitis is an acute or chronic inflammation of the tonsils, the glandular tissue near the back of the tongue that is part of the body's natural defense system. Tonsillitis usually develops suddenly because of streptococcal infection, although it can also be caused by viral infections. It is typically accompanied by sore throat, fever, chills, headache, poor appetite, and weakness. The tonsils become swollen and red, and streaks of pus are often visible on the surface.

Acute tonsillitis usually clears up in about a week, but antibiotics may be needed to prevent complications like middle-ear and sinus infections. In chronic tonsillitis, the tonsils tend to become inflamed episodically during periods of acute infection. Tonsillitis is more common in children than in adults.

Herbs to Consider for Tonsillitis

Herbs known as *lymphatic alteratives* are considered to be specifically indicated for tonsillitis. The most relevant is cleavers.

Tonsillitis Tincture

This formula offers antimicrobial, immune-boosting herbs along with cleavers, which is specifically indicated for tonsillitis.

2 parts cleavers
2 parts echinacea
1 part wild indigo
1 part calendula

To make: Combine herbs with alcohol to make a tincture, as described on page 115.
To use: Take 5 ml of the tincture three times daily.

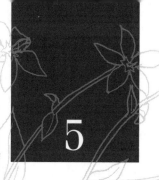

A GUIDE TO
THE HEALING HERBS

Different conditions of the digestive system produce common processes, symptoms, and general experiences. Knowing herbal approaches that will address these general patterns helps the herbalist treat a specific disease.

The following *materia medica,* or listing of herbs used to make medicine, offers a guide to the primary actions and uses for the herbs of particular relevance for the respiratory system. You will find many of these herbs available at an herb shop, natural food store, or through a mail-order supplier of bulk herbs.

ANISEED *(Pimpinella anisum)*

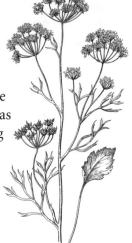

Part used: Seed.
Actions: Expectorant, antispasmodic, carminative, antimicrobial, aromatic, galactogogue.
Indications: The volatile oil in aniseed helps ease gripe, intestinal colic, and flatulence. It also has expectorant and antispasmodic actions, making it useful against bronchitis. It may be used for tracheitis when persistent irritable coughing is present and for whooping cough. Externally,

the oil may be added to an ointment for treating scabies. The oil by itself will help control lice. Aniseed has been shown to increase mucociliary transport, and this supports its use as an expectorant. It has mild estrogenic effects.

Preparation and Dosage: To make an infusion, gently crush the seeds to release the volatile oil. Pour 1 cup (240 ml) boiling water over 1–2 teaspoons seeds. Let stand, covered, 5–10 minutes. Drink 1 cup (240 ml) three times a day. To treat flatulence, drink the tea slowly before meals.

When taking oil internally, add 1 drop oil to ½ teaspoon (2 ml) honey.

BALM OF GILEAD *(Populus × jackii 'Gileadensis')*

Part used: Closed buds.

Actions: Stimulating expectorant, antimicrobial, vulnerary.

Indications: Balm of Gilead soothes, disinfects, and acts as an astringent on the mucous membranes, making it an excellent remedy for sore throats, coughs, and laryngitis. It's specifically indicated for laryngitis accompanied by voice loss. It may be used in chronic bronchitis. Externally, it can be used to ease inflammations caused by rheumatism and arthritis and to treat dry and scaly skin conditions, like psoriasis and dry eczema.

Preparation and Dosage: To make an infusion, pour 1 cup (240 ml) boiling water over 1 teaspoon buds; let infuse 10–15 minutes. Drink three times daily or more — if you can deal with the taste!

When using a tincture, take 1–2 ml three times daily.

BLOODROOT *(Sanguinaria canadensis)*

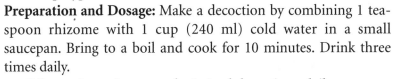

Part used: Rhizome, dried.

Actions: Expectorant, antispasmodic, emetic, cathartic, nervine, cardioactive, topical irritant.

Indications: Bloodroot is mainly used to treat bronchitis. Its stimulating properties make it useful as an emetic and expectorant, but it also relaxes the bronchial muscles. As a result, it's helpful against asthma, croup, and laryngitis. It's superb for chronic congestive conditions of the lungs, including bronchitis, emphysema, and bronchiectasis. It acts as a stimulant in cases of deficient peripheral circulation. It may be used as a snuff in the treatment of nasal polyps.

Preparation and Dosage: Make a decoction by combining 1 teaspoon rhizome with 1 cup (240 ml) cold water in a small saucepan. Bring to a boil and cook for 10 minutes. Drink three times daily.

When using a tincture, take 1–2 ml three times daily.

CAUTION!

Bloodroot should not be used by children. It should not be used during pregnancy or lactation. Long-term use has been linked to glaucoma. Large internal doses can cause vomiting, fainting, paralysis, and collapse.

BONESET *(Eupatorium perfoliatum)*

Parts used: Leaves and flowers, dried.

Actions: Diaphoretic, bitter, laxative, tonic, antispasmodic, carminative, astringent.

Indications: Boneset is one of the best remedies for the relief of flu symptoms. It quickly relieves aches and pains and helps the body deal with fever. It can help clear the upper respiratory tract of mucus congestion. Its mild aperient activity will ease constipation. It may be used safely for fever and as a general cleansing agent. It may provide symptomatic aid in the treatment of muscular rheumatism.

Preparation and Dosage: To make an infusion, pour 1 cup (240 ml) boiling water over 1–2 teaspoons dried herbs; let infuse 10–15 minutes. Drink as hot as possible every 30 minutes.

When using a tincture, take 2–4 ml three times a day.

CALENDULA *(Calendula officinalis)*

Parts used: Petals, flower heads.

Actions: Anti-inflammatory, antispasmodic, lymphatic, astringent, vulnerary, emmenagogue, antimicrobial.

Indications: Calendula is one of the best herbs for treating local skin problems, including those caused by infection or physical damage (for example, abrasions). It may be used for external bleeding, bruises, or strains. It's also helpful for slow-healing wounds and skin ulcers and is ideal for treating minor burns and scalds. It may be used topically in lotions, poultices, or compresses.

Internally, calendula is valuable against digestive inflammation. It may be used to treat gastric and duodenal ulcers. As a cholagogue, it helps relieve gallbladder problems and indigestion. Externally, it can be used as a lotion or ointment for cuts, bruises, diaper rash, sore nipples, burns, and scalds.

Calendula has marked antifungal activity and may be used internally and externally to combat fungal infections. As an emmenagogue, it has a reputation for helping with delayed menstruation and painful periods.

Preparation and Dosage: To make an infusion, pour 1 cup (240 ml) boiling water over 1–2 teaspoons florets; let infuse 10–15 minutes. Drink three times a day.

When using a tincture, take 1–4 ml three times a day.

CAYENNE (*Capsicum* species)

Part used: Fruit.
Actions: Stimulant, carminative, anticatarrhal, sialagogue, rubefacient, antimicrobial.
Indications: Cayenne is the most useful of the systemic stimulants. It stimulates blood flow and strengthens the heart, arteries, capillaries, and nerves. A general tonic, it is specific for both the circulatory and digestive systems. It may be used for flatulent dyspepsia and colic, as well as for cold hands and feet caused by insufficient peripheral circulation. It's helpful for general debility and for warding off colds.

Externally, cayenne is used as a rubefacient for problems like lumbago and rheumatic pains. As an ointment, it helps unbroken chilblains as long as it's used in moderation. As a gargle for laryngitis, it combines well with myrrh. The combination of cayenne and myrrh also makes a good antiseptic wash.

Preparation and Dosage: To make an infusion, pour 1 cup (240 ml) boiling water over ½–1 teaspoon dried herb; let infuse 10 minutes. Mix 1 tablespoon (15 ml) of the infusion with hot water and drink as needed.

When using a tincture, take 0.25–1 ml three times a day or as needed.

Contraindications: Cayenne may cause eye and skin irritation.

CLEAVERS *(Galium aparine)*

Parts used: Dried aerial parts and freshly expressed juice.

Actions: Diuretic, alterative, anti-inflammatory, tonic, astringent.

Indications: Cleavers is very valuable and may be the best tonic for the lymphatic system. It may be used safely for a wide range of problems, including swollen glands (lymphadenitis) anywhere in the body. It's especially good for tonsillitis and adenoid trouble. It is helpful in skin conditions, particularly those that are dry (like psoriasis). It is useful in the treatment of cystitis and other urinary conditions accompanied by pain; for this purpose, it may be combined with urinary demulcents. Cleavers has traditionally been used to treat ulcers and tumors, perhaps because of its effects on lymphatic drainage, which helps detoxify tissue. Cleavers also makes an excellent vegetable.

Preparation and Dosage: To make an infusion, pour 1 cup (240 ml) boiling water over 2–3 teaspoons dried herb; let infuse 10–15 minutes. Drink three times a day.

When using a tincture, take 2–4 ml three times a day.

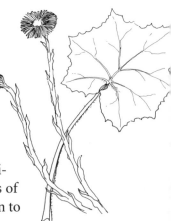

COLTSFOOT *(Tussilago farfara)*

Parts used: Flowers and leaves, dried.

Actions: Expectorant, antitussive, antispasmodic, demulcent, anti-catarrhal, diuretic.

Indications: Coltsfoot combines a soothing expectorant effect with an antispasmodic action. There are useful levels of zinc in the leaves, which have been shown to have marked anti-inflammatory effects. Coltsfoot may be used in chronic or acute bronchitis, irritating coughs, whooping coughs, and asthma. Because of its soothing expectorant action, coltsfoot can be used to relieve most respiratory conditions, including chronic emphysema. As a mild diuretic, it has been used in cystitis. The fresh bruised leaves can be applied to boils, abscesses, and suppurating ulcers.

Preparation and Dosage: To make an infusion, pour 1 cup (240 ml) boiling water over 1–2 teaspoons dried flowers or leaves; let infuse 10 minutes. Drink three times a day, as hot as possible.

When using a tincture, take 2–4 ml three times a day.

Contraindications: Avoid excessive or long-term use of coltsfoot. Do not use this herb during pregnancy or lactation. It may cause liver damage.

COMFREY *(Symphytum officinale)*

Parts used: Root, rhizome, and leaves.

Actions: Vulnerary, demulcent, anti-inflammatory, astringent, expectorant.

Indications: The impressive wound-healing properties of comfrey are partly due to the presence of allantoin. This chemical stimulates cell proliferation and augments wound healing inside and out. Because comfrey contains substantial demulcent mucilage, it's a powerful healing agent for gastric and duodenal ulcers, hiatal hernia, and ulcerative colitis. Its astringency helps hemorrhages wherever they occur.

In the respiratory system, comfrey is helpful against bronchitis and irritable cough because it soothes and reduces irritation while aiding expectoration. It may be used externally to speed wound healing and to guard against incorrect development of scar tissue. Care should be taken with very deep wounds, however, because the external application of comfrey can cause tissue to form over the wound before it has healed deeply, and this may lead to abscesses. Comfrey may be applied as a compress or poultice for external ulcers, wounds, or fractures. It's excellent for chronic varicose ulcers and is thought to have an anticancer action.

Combinations: For gastric ulcers and inflammations, comfrey combines well with marsh mallow and meadowsweet. For chest and bronchial troubles, use comfrey with coltsfoot, white horehound, or elecampane. For wound healing, use comfrey with calendula.

Preparation and Dosage: To make a decoction, put 1–3 teaspoons dried herb in 1 cup (240 ml) water. Bring to a boil and let simmer 10–15 minutes. Drink three times a day.

When using a tincture, take 2–4 ml three times a day.

Contraindications: Comfrey should not be used by pregnant women or people with liver problems.

COWSLIP *(Primula veris)*

Part used: Flower heads, fresh or dried.

Actions: Expectorant, astringent.

Indications: Cowslip is useful for treating any condition accompanied by coughs and catarrh. It has a reputation for being helpful in arthritis, rheumatism, and liver and kidney problems. Because of its astringency, it is useful for diarrhea.

Preparation and Dosage: To make an infusion, pour 1 cup (240 ml) boiling water over 1 teaspoon dried herb; let infuse 10 minutes. Drink three or four times a day.

When using a tincture, take 2–4 ml three times a day.

ECHINACEA *(Echinacea species)*

Part used: Root.

Actions: Antimicrobial, immunomodulator, anticatarrhal, alterative.

Indications: Echinacea is one of the primary antimicrobials. It is often effective against bacterial as well as viral attacks. It may be used for boils, septicemia, and similar infections. Used in conjunction with other herbs, it's helpful for treating infections anywhere in the body.

Echinacea is especially useful for infections of the upper respiratory tract, such as laryngitis and tonsillitis. It's also used for catarrhal conditions of the nose and sinuses. Tinctures or decoctions may be used as mouthwashes for treating pyorrhea and gingivitis. It may be used as an external lotion to help septic sores and cuts.

Much research has been done on echinacea, and these studies have provided important insights into the herb's activity and potential uses. Glycosides from the roots have mild activity against streptococci and *Staphylococcus aureus*. The tincture has been shown to reduce both the rate of growth and the rate of reproduction of *Trichomonas vaginalis*. Echinacea was found to be effective in halting the recurrence of *Candida albicans* infection.

Preparation and Dosage: To make a decoction, put 1–2 teaspoons root in 1 cup (240 ml) water. Slowly bring to a boil, then let simmer 10–15 minutes. Drink three times a day.

When using a tincture, take 1–4 ml three times a day.

ELDER *(Sambucus nigra)*

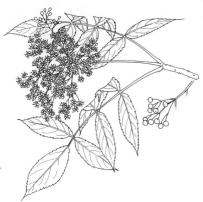

Parts used: Bark, flowers, berries, leaves.

Actions:

Bark: purgative, emetic, diuretic.

Leaves: used externally, emollient and vulnerary; used internally, purgative, expectorant, diuretic, diaphoretic

Flowers: diaphoretic, anticatarrhal, antispasmodic

Berries: diaphoretic, diuretic, laxative

Indications: The elder tree is a medicine chest in itself. The leaves are used for bruises, sprains, wounds, and chilblains. It has been reported that elder leaves may be helpful in an ointment used for tumors. Elderflower leaves and flowers are ideal for the treatment of colds and the flu. In fact, they're helpful for any catarrhal inflammation of the upper respiratory tract, such as that caused by hay fever and sinusitis. Catarrhal deafness responds well to elderflower. Elderberries have properties similar to those of elderflowers and are also useful for treating rheumatism.

Preparation and Dosage: To make an infusion, pour 1 cup (240 ml) boiling water over 2 teaspoons dried or fresh blossoms; let infuse 10 minutes. Drink hot three times a day.

To make a juice, boil fresh berries in water for 2–3 minutes, then express the juice. To preserve, add 1 part honey to 10 parts juice; bring to a boil, then let cool. To use, dilute in hot water and drink 1 glass twice a day.

To make an ointment, combine 3 parts fresh elder leaves with 6 parts melted petroleum jelly; heat until the leaves are crisp. Strain and store.

When using a tincture, take 2–4 ml three times a day.

Contraindications: The leaves and bark of elder are poisonous and should be used only as directed.

ELECAMPANE *(Inula helenium)*

Part used: Rhizome.
Actions: Expectorant, antitussive, diaphoretic, hepatic, antimicrobial.
Indications: Elecampane is specifically indicated for irritating bronchial coughs, especially in children. It may be used whenever there is copious catarrh, as in bronchitis or emphysema.

Elecampane provides a good illustration of the complex and integrated ways in which herbs work. The mucilage has a relaxing effect, and the essential oils are stimulating. This combination results in a soothing action accompanied by antibacterial effects.

Elecampane may be used for asthma and bronchitic asthma. It has been used in the treatment of tuberculosis. The bitter principle makes it helpful for stimulating digestion and appetite.

Preparation and Dosage: To make an infusion, pour 1 cup cold water (240 ml) over 1 teaspoon shredded root; let stand for 8–10 hours. Reheat and drink very hot three times a day.

When using a tincture, take 1–2 ml three times a day.

Contraindications: Do not use elecampagne during pregnancy or lactation.

EYEBRIGHT *(Euphrasia officinalis)*

Parts used: Dried aerial parts.

Actions: Anticatarrhal, astringent, anti-inflammatory.

Indications: Eyebright is an excellent remedy for problems affecting the mucous membranes. Its combination of anti-inflammatory and astringent properties makes it appropriate for many conditions. Internally, it's a powerful anticatarrhal and is therefore useful for nasal catarrh, sinusitis, and other congestive conditions. It's best known for its use in conditions of the eye. It can help relieve acute or chronic inflammations, stinging and weeping eyes, and oversensitivity to light. Used as a compress and internally, it's valuable for conjunctivitis and blepharitis.

Preparation and Dosage: To make an infusion, pour 1 cup (240 ml) boiling water over 1 teaspoon dried herb; let infuse 5–10 minutes. Drink three times a day.

To make a compress, place 1 teaspoon dried herb in 1 pint (500 ml) water. Boil 10 minutes, then cool slightly. Moisten a compress (cotton, wool, gauze, or muslin) in the liquid, wring it out, and place it over the eyes for 15 minutes. Repeat several times a day.

When using a tincture, take 1–4 ml three times a day.

GARLIC *(Allium sativum)*

Part used: Bulb.

Actions: Antimicrobial, diaphoretic, chola-gogue, hypotensive, antispasmodic.

Indications: Garlic aids and supports the body in ways that no other herb does. One of the most effective antimicrobial plants avail-able, it acts on bacteria, viruses, and alimen-tary parasites. The volatile oil is an effective agent that is largely secreted through the lungs. Because of this, it's effective for treating chronic bronchitis, respiratory catarrh, and recur-rent colds and flu. It may be helpful in the treat-ment of whooping cough and, as part of a broader approach, bronchitic asthma. In general, it may be used to prevent most digestive and respiratory infectious conditions. It's especially good for digestive problems because it supports the development of the natural bacterial flora while killing pathogenic organisms.

Garlic has an international reputation for lowering high blood pressure and blood cholesterol levels and improving the health of the cardiovascular system. It should be thought of as a basic food that will augment the body's health and provide gen-eral protection.

Combinations: For microbial infections, garlic combines well with echinacea.

Preparation and Dosage: Eat 1 clove of garlic three times a day. If the smell becomes a problem, substitute garlic oil capsules three times daily.

GOLDENROD *(Solidago species)*

Parts used: Aerial parts, dried.

Actions: Anticatarrhal, anti-inflammatory, antimicrobial, astrin-gent, diaphoretic, carminative, diuretic.

Indications: Goldenrod is probably the first plant you should think of when you need to treat upper respiratory catarrh, whether acute or chronic. It may be used in combination with other herbs for flu. Its carminative properties are helpful for flatulent dyspepsia. As an anti-inflammatory urinary antiseptic, goldenrod may be used for cystitis, urethritis, and similar conditions. It can be used to promote the healing of wounds. As a gargle, it can be used to treat laryngitis and pharyngitis.

Preparation and Dosage: To make an infusion, pour 1 cup (240 ml) boiling water over 2–3 teaspoons dried herb; let infuse 10–15 minutes. Drink three times a day or use infusion as a gargle three times a day. When using a tincture, take 2–4 ml three times a day.

GOLDENSEAL (Hydrastis canadensis)

Parts used: Root and rhizome.

Actions: Bitter, hepatic, alterative, anticatarrhal, antimicrobial, anti-inflammatory, astringent, laxative, expectorant, emmenagogue, oxytocic.

Indications: Goldenseal is a very useful remedy because of its tonic effects on the mucous membranes of the body. It's useful for treating all digestive problems, from peptic ulcer to colitis. Its bitter stimulation helps in loss of appetite, and its alkaloids stimulate bile production and secretion.

All catarrhal conditions, especially sinus conditions, improve with goldenseal. Goldenseal's antimicrobial properties seem to be related to the alkaloids it contains. For example, goldenseal contains a constituent called *berberine*, which has antibiotic, immunostimulatory, antispasmodic, sedative, hypotensive, uterotonic, choleretic, and carminative activity.

Contraindications

Goldenseal should not be used by pregnant women before labor begins.

Although berberine is not in the same league as antibiotics, it has a broad spectrum of antimicrobial activity. Its in vitro antimicrobial effects have been demonstrated against bacteria, protozoa, and fungi, and its action against some pathogens is actually stronger than that of common antibiotics. (It's important to remember, however, that herbal medicine depends on the use of whole plants and not single extracted constituents.) Because berberine inhibits *Candida* species, along with other organisms, it can help prevent the overgrowth of yeast — a common side effect of antibiotic use.

> ### Note
> Goldenseal is an endangered plant, and consumers should make every effort to buy material that has been cultivated. Products made from material collected in the wild should not be purchased unless labeled as "ethically wildcrafted."

This fascinating alkaloid increases blood supply to the spleen. It has also been shown to activate macrophages in numerous ways. It can inhibit tumor formation in the laboratory and may have antineoplastic activity.

Several clinical studies have shown that berberine stimulates the secretion of bile and bilirubin. One clinical trial examined the effect of berberine on 225 patients with chronic cholecystitis. Over 24 to 48 hours, oral doses of 5 to 20 mg taken three times a day before meals resolved clinical symptoms, decreased bilirubin levels, and increased the bile volume of the gallbladder.

Traditionally, goldenseal has been used during labor to strengthen contractions. It should be avoided in pregnancy until labor begins. Applied externally, it can be helpful in treating eczema, ringworm, itching, earache, and conjunctivitis.

Preparation and Dosage: To make an infusion, pour 1 cup (240 ml) boiling water over ½–1 teaspoon powdered herb; let infuse 10–15 minutes. Drink three times a day.

When using a tincture, take 1 ml three times a day.

GRINDELIA (*Grindelia* species)

Parts used: Leaves and flowers, dried.
Actions: Antispasmodic, expectorant, hypotensive.
Indications: Grindelia relaxes both smooth and cardiac muscles. This helps explain its use in the treatment of asthmatic and bronchial conditions, especially those associated with a rapid heartbeat and nervous response. Because of its relaxing effect on the heart and pulse rate, grindelia may reduce blood pressure. Externally, lotion made from the herb is used to treat dermatitis caused by poison ivy.
Preparation and Dosage: To make an infusion, pour 1 cup (240 ml) boiling water over 1 teaspoon dried herb; let infuse 10–15 minutes. Drink three times a day.

When using a tincture, take 1–2 ml three times a day.

HOREHOUND (*Marrubium vulgare*)

Parts used: Leaves and flowering tops, dried.
Actions: Expectorant, antispasmodic, bitter, vulnerary, emmenagogue.
Indications: Horehound is valuable in the treatment of bronchitis accompanied by a non-productive cough. It relaxes the smooth muscles of the bronchi while promoting mucus production and expectoration. It can be beneficial in the treatment of whooping cough. The bitter action stimulates the flow and secretion of bile from the gallbladder, aiding digestion. Horehound is used externally to promote wound healing.
Preparation and Dosage: To make an infusion, pour 1 cup (240 ml) boiling water over ½–1 teaspoon dried herb; let infuse 10–15 minutes. Drink three times a day.

When using a tincture, take 1–2 ml three times a day.
Contraindications: Do not use horehound during pregnancy.

Hyssop *(Hyssopus officinalis)*

Parts used: Leaves and flowers, dried.
Actions: Antispasmodic, expectorant, diaphoretic, nervine, anti-inflammatory, carminative, hepatic, emmenagogue.
Indications: Hyssop has an interesting range of uses that are largely due to the antispasmodic action of its volatile oil. It's used to treat coughs, bronchitis, and chronic catarrh. Its diaphoretic properties make it useful against the common cold. As a nervine, it may be used to relieve anxiety, hysteria, and petit mal (a form of epilepsy).
Preparation and Dosage: To make an infusion, pour 1 cup (240 ml) boiling water over 1–2 teaspoons dried herb; let infuse 10–15 minutes. Drink three times a day.

When using a tincture, take 1–4 ml three times a day.
Contraindications: Do not use hyssop during pregnancy.

Iceland Moss *(Cetraria islandica)*

Part used: Entire plant, fresh or dried.
Actions: Demulcent, anti-inflammatory, antiemetic, expectorant.
Indications: As a soothing demulcent with a high mucilage content, Iceland moss can be helpful for treating gastritis, vomiting, and dyspepsia. It is often used in respiratory catarrh and bronchitis because of its soothing effect on mucous membranes. Its nourishing qualities contribute to the treatment of cachexia, a state of malnourishment and debility.
Preparation and Dosage: To make a decoction, put 1 teaspoon shredded moss in 1 cup (240 ml) cold water. Boil 3 minutes, then

let stand 10 minutes. Drink 1 cup (240 ml) in the morning and evening.

When using a tincture, take 1–2 ml three times a day.

IPECACUANHA *(Cephaëlis ipecacuanha)*

Part used: Rhizome, dried.
Actions: Expectorant, sialagogue, antiprotozoal.
Indications: Ipecacuanha is mainly used as an expectorant in treating bronchitis and other conditions, like whooping cough. At higher doses, it is a powerful emetic and can be used to treat poisoning. Just as ipecac aids expectoration by stimulating mucus secretion and removal, ipecacuanha stimulates production of saliva. It has been found to be effective in the treatment of amoebic dysentery.
Preparation and Dosage: Because ipecacuanha is so powerful, only a very small amount should be used. To make an infusion, use 0.01–0.25 g herb, an amount about the size of a pea. Pour 1 cup boiling water (240 ml) over the herb; let infuse 5 minutes. Drink three times a day.
Contraindications: Ipecacuanha should not be used by people with heart disease or people who are generally weakened (for example, through shock or disability).

IRISH MOSS *(Chondrus crispus)*

Part used: Entire plant, fresh or dried.
Actions: Expectorant, demulcent, anti-inflammatory.
Indications: With all of the recent attention given to dramatically effective "miracle drugs," it is refreshing to remember the nourishing and strengthening abilities of herbs like Irish moss. Because Irish moss is very safe, it can be used for many conditions.

Irish moss has traditionally been used to treat respiratory illnesses, such as irritating coughs, bronchitis, and various lung problems. When a demulcent is called for, Irish moss may be used for digestive conditions, like gastritis and ulceration of the stomach and duodenum. Its soothing activity helps relieve inflammations of the urinary system. At one time, it was used much as corn silk is used today. Irish moss has even been used as a food in maintenance diets for diabetic patients.

Irish moss is primarily used to speed recuperation from debilitating illnesses, especially tuberculosis and pneumonia. With degenerative diseases becoming the major killers in our society, herbs such as Irish moss and other tonic nutritive remedies offer hope and should be explored more fully.

Preparation and Dosage: When using fresh Irish moss as a food, wash it well. Add 1 cup (240 ml) herb to 3 cups (720 ml) milk or water, and flavor to taste. Simmer slowly until most of the herb has dissolved. Remove any undissolved fragments, then pour into a mold to set.

To make a decoction using dried herb, steep ½ ounce (15 g) herb in cold water for 15 minutes. Then boil 10–15 minutes in 3 pints (1.5 L) water or milk. Strain and drink. The decoction is often combined with licorice, lemon, ginger, or cinnamon and may be sweetened to taste.

LICORICE *(Glycyrrhiza glabra)*

Part used: Root, dried.

Actions: Expectorant, demulcent, anti-inflammatory, antihepatotoxic, antispasmodic, mild laxative.

Indications: Licorice is a traditional herbal remedy that has an ancient history and is used worldwide. Modern research shows that it affects the endocrine system and the liver and other organs. Licorice contains constituents that are metabolized in the body to form molecules whose structures are similar to those of the adrenal cortex hormones. This may explain the herb's anti-inflammatory action.

As an antihepatotoxic agent, licorice can be effective in the treatment of chronic hepatitis and cirrhosis (it has been widely used for this purpose in Japan). Most liver-oriented research has focused on the triterpene glycyrrhizin, which inhibits hepatocyte injury caused by carbon tetrachloride, benzene hexachloride, and PCB (polychlorobenzenes). Antibody production is enhanced by glycyrrhizin, possibly through the production of interleukin.

Glycyrrhizin inhibits the growth of several DNA and RNA viruses and irreversibly inactivates *Herpes simplex* virus particles. It has a wide range of uses in bronchial problems, including catarrh, bronchitis, and coughs, and is used in allopathic medicine as a treatment for peptic ulceration. Herbalists also use it to treat gastritis and ulcers. It can be used to relieve abdominal colic.

Preparation and Dosage: To make a decoction, put ½–1 teaspoon root in 1 cup (240 ml) water. Bring to a boil and simmer 10–15 minutes. Drink three times a day.

When using a tincture, take 1–3 ml three times a day.

CAUTION!

There is a small possibility that licorice, used in large doses, may affect the body's electrolyte balance. It should not be used by people with congestive heart failure, diabetes, glaucoma, edema, hypertension, or kidney disease. It should not be used by people taking the prescription drug digoxin. Do not use during pregnancy. Avoid prolonged use, which can promote high blood pressure, cardiovascular toxicity, and edema.

LOBELIA (*Lobelia inflata*)

Parts used: Aerial parts.

Actions: Antiasthmatic, antispasmodic, expectorant, emetic, nervine.

Indications: Lobelia is one of the most useful systemic relaxants available. It has a general depressant action on the central and autonomic nervous system and on neuromuscular action. It is used to treat many conditions, often in combination with other herbs. Its primary specific use is for bronchitic asthma and bronchitis. Analysis of the action of its alkaloids has revealed apparently paradoxical effects. Lobeline is a powerful respiratory stimulant, and isolobelanine is an emetic and respiratory relaxant. The herb will stimulate catarrhal secretion and expectoration while relaxing the muscles of the respiratory system. The overall action is a truly holistic combination of stimulation and relaxation.

Preparation and Dosage: To make an infusion, pour 1 cup (240 ml) boiling water over ¼–½ teaspoon of dried leaves; let infuse 10–15 minutes. Drink three times a day.

When using a tincture, take ½ ml three times a day.

CAUTION!

Do not use lobelia during pregnancy. May cause nausea and vomiting.

LUNGWORT (*Pulmonaria officinalis*)

Part used: Leaves and flowers, dried.

Actions: Demulcent, expectorant, astringent, anti-inflammatory, vulnerary.

Indications: Lungwort can be used in two broad areas. As its name suggests, it's commonly used in the treatment of coughs and cases of bronchitis, especially

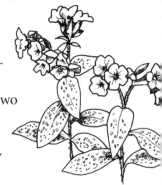

those associated with upper respiratory catarrh. The other area of use is related to the herb's astringency. It's helpful for treating diarrhea, especially in children, and for easing hemorrhoids. It may be used externally to help heal cuts and wounds.

Preparation and Dosage: To make an infusion, pour 1 cup (240 ml) boiling water over 1–2 teaspoons dried herb; let infuse 10–15 minutes. Drink three times a day.

When using a tincture, take 1–4 ml three times a day.

Ma Huang (Ephedra sinica)

Part used: Aerial stems.

Actions: Vasodilator, hypertensive, circulatory stimulant, antiallergic.

Indications: Ma huang has been used in China for at least 5,000 years to treat a range of health problems, especially in the respiratory system. This ancient medicinal plant was also mentioned in the Hindu Vedas (ancient holy writings). With the discovery of the alkaloids in ma huang, traditional herbal wisdom has been verified and modern medicine has been given important healing tools.

Many therapeutically active alkaloids are found in Ma Huang *Ephedra*; they sometimes amount to 2 percent of the dried herb. The alkaloids were first isolated in 1887 and came into extensive use in the 1930s. Various species of Asian *Ephedra* are a source of the widely used alkaloids ephedrine and pseudoephedrine. The alkaloids in *Ephedra* apparently have opposite effects on the body. The overall action, however, is one of balance and benefit. A brief review of the pharmacology of these alkaloids might be illuminating. Ephedrine was the first ma huang alkaloid to find wide use in Western medicine and was hailed as a "cure" for asthma because of its ability to relax the airways in the lungs. Unfortunately, as is often the case with "miracle cures," it soon became clear that this isolated constituent of *Ephedra* had unacceptable side effects that dramatically limited its use. Ephedrine stimulated the autonomic nervous system, causing, among other things, high blood pressure.

When studies were done using the whole plant, only a small blood pressure elevation was found. This led to the discovery that pseudoephedrine, another of the alkaloids present, slightly reduces both heart rate and lowers blood pressure, eliminating the side effects that often accompany the use of ephedrine. Pseudo-ephedrine is an effective bronchodilator that is as strong as ephedrine but is less stimulating to the nervous system. It results in fewer episodes of vasoconstriction, tachycardia (heart palpitations), and other cardiovascular symptoms.

Clinical studies have found that pseudoephedrine has insignificant side effects. The U.S. Food and Drug Administration recognizes its efficacy and safety and has approved its use in over-the-counter medications as a safe and effective nasal decongestant. In practice, the natural form is better tolerated and has less effect on the heart. The naturally occurring alkaloids have been synthesized in the laboratory, however, even though they have the same molecular structure, they have different physical properties. The natural form rotates polarized light to the left, while the synthetic form is optically inactive.

All of these findings validate the traditional use of *Ephedra sinica* as a safe, effective treatment for nasal congestion and sinus

---

CAUTION!

Ma huang should not be used by people with cardiovascular conditions, high blood pressure, heart disease, gastric ulcers, glaucoma, anxiety disorders, thyroid disease, or diabetes. Should not be used by men who have trouble urinating because of prostate enlargement. Should not be used during pregnancy or lactation. Should not be used by people taking monoamine oxidase (MAO) inhibitors. Do not exceed the recommended dosage. Do not combine with caffeine. For short-term use only.

pressure. The herb is very useful for asthma and associated conditions (for example, bronchial asthma, bronchitis, and whooping cough) because it can relieve spasms in the bronchial tubes. It also reduces allergic reactions, so it has a role in the treatment of hay fever and other allergies. It may be used to treat low blood pressure and circulatory insufficiency.

Preparation and Dosage: To make a decoction, put 1–2 teaspoons dried herb in 1 cup (240 ml) water. Bring to a boil and simmer 10–15 minutes. Drink three times a day.

When using a tincture, take 1–4 ml three times a day.

MARSH MALLOW *(Althaea officinalis)*

Parts used: Root, leaf.

Actions: Demulcent, emollient, diuretic, anti-inflammatory, expectorant.

Indications: Marsh mallow's abundance of mucilage makes it an excellent demulcent. The roots are used mainly for treating the digestive system; the leaves are used more for the urinary system and the lungs.

Marsh mallow helps all inflammatory conditions of the gastrointestinal tract. It can be used to treat inflammations of the mouth as well as gastritis, peptic ulceration, and colitis. The leaves are helpful for treating cystitis, urethritis, and urinary gravel, as well as bronchitis, respiratory catarrh, and irritating coughs. Externally, marsh mallow is often used in "drawing" ointments for the treatment of abscesses and boils. It's also used as an emollient for varicose veins and ulcers.

Preparation and Dosage: Make a cold infusion with marsh mallow roots by adding 2–4 g root to 1 cup (240 ml) cold water. Let infuse overnight, then drink.

When using a tincture, take 1–4 ml three times a day.

MOTHERWORT *(Leonurus cardiaca)*

Parts used: Aerial parts.

Actions: Nervine, emmenagogue, antispasmodic, hepatic, cardiac tonic, hypotensive.

Indications: This herb is often used to treat menstrual and uterine conditions. It's a useful, relaxing tonic for menopausal changes. It may be used to ease false labor pains. It's an excellent tonic for the heart because it strengthens without straining. It's specifically indicated for tachycardia (heart palpitations), especially when anxiety is involved. Motherwort may be used in all heart conditions that are associated with anxiety and tension. Chinese research suggests that this herb will reduce blood platelet aggregation and decrease blood lipid levels.

Preparation and Dosage: To make an infusion, pour 1 cup (240 ml) boiling water over 1–2 teaspoons dried herb; let infuse 10–15 minutes. Drink three times a day.

When using the tincture, take 1–4 ml three times a day.

Contraindications: Can cause skin irritation in some people. Do not use during pregnancy.

MULLEIN *(Verbascum thapsus)*

Parts used: Leaves and flowers, dried.

Actions: Expectorant, demulcent, diuretic, anti-inflammatory, nervine, antispasmodic, vulnerary, alterative, astringent.

Indications: Mullein is very beneficial for most conditions that affect the respiratory system. It is ideal for toning the mucous membranes of the respiratory system and for reducing inflammation while stimulating fluid production and promoting expectoration.

Mullein is specifically indicated for bronchitis that's accompanied by a hard cough and soreness. Its anti-inflammatory and demulcent properties make it useful against inflammation of the trachea and associated conditions. Externally, it can be used as an extract made with olive oil to soothe and heal any inflamed surface or to ease ear problems.

Preparation and Dosage: To make an infusion, pour 1 cup (240 ml) boiling water over 1–2 teaspoons dried leaves or flowers; let infuse 10–15 minutes. Drink three times a day.

When using a tincture, take 1–4 ml three times a day.

Contraindications: Mullein is not intended for repeated long-term use.

MUSTARD *(Sinapis alba and Brassica nigra)*

Part used: Seed.

Actions: Rubefacient, irritant, stimulant, diuretic, emetic.

Indications: This well-known spice is mainly used as an external stimulant. The rubefacient action mildly irritates the skin, which stimulates circulation in the area and relieves muscular and skeletal pain. Mustard's stimulating diaphoretic action is similar to that of cayenne and ginger. For relieving fever, colds, and the flu, mustard may be used as a tea or ground and sprinkled into a bath. Because it stimulates circulation, it can be helpful for treating chilblains. An infusion or poultice of mustard may be used to ease bronchitis.

Preparation and Dosage: To make a poultice, mix 100 g freshly ground seeds with warm water to form a thick paste. Spread the paste on a piece of cloth the size of the area that needs to be covered. (To prevent the paste from sticking to the skin, put a damp piece of gauze between skin and poultice.) Apply the poultice and remove after 1 minute. The skin may be slightly irritated by this treatment; you can relieve the irritation by applying olive oil afterward.

To make an infusion, pour 1 cup (240 ml) boiling water over 1 teaspoon mustard flour; let infuse 5 minutes. Drink the infusion three times a day.

To prepare a foot bath, make an infusion by pouring 2 pints (1 L) boiling water over 1 tablespoon bruised seeds.

MYRRH (Commiphora molmol)

Part used: Gum resin.

Actions: Antimicrobial, astringent, carminative, anticatarrhal, expectorant, vulnerary.

Indications: Myrrh is an effective antimicrobial agent that has been shown to work in two complementary ways. Primarily, it stimulates the production of white blood cells, which have antipathogenic actions. It also has a direct antimicrobial effect. It can be used for a wide variety of conditions that involve infection, including mouth ulcers, gingivitis, and pyorrhea. Myrrh has anticatarrhal properties and can be used to relieve pharyngitis and sinusitis. It's also used to treat laryngitis and other respiratory problems. Systemically, it can be used to treat boils and similar conditions, along with glandular fever, brucellosis, and (when combined with other remedies) the common cold. Externally, it acts as an antiseptic and helps speed healing of wounds and abrasions.

Preparation and Dosage: It's difficult to dissolve myrrh in water, so powder it well when making an infusion. Pour 1 cup (240 ml) boiling water over 1–2 teaspoons powder; let infuse 10–15 minutes. Drink three times a day.

When using a tincture, take 1–4 ml three times a day.

Contraindications: Do not use myrrh during pregnancy.

NETTLE *(Urtica dioica)*

Parts used: Aerial parts.

Actions: Astringent, diuretic, tonic, hypotensive.

Indications: Nettle is an extremely versatile herb that strengthens and supports the whole body. It's used in Europe as a spring tonic and general detoxifying remedy. In some cases of rheumatism and arthritis, it can be astoundingly successful. It's specifically indicated for cases of childhood eczema and is especially useful for nervous eczema. As an astringent, it may be used for nose-bleeds or other types of bleeding, including bleeding that occurs internally, as in uterine hemorrhage.

Preparation and Dosage: To make an infusion, pour 1 cup (240 ml) boiling water over 1–3 teaspoons dried herb; let infuse 10–15 minutes. Drink three times a day.

When using a tincture, take 1–4 ml three times a day.

Contraindications: The fresh herb contains stinging hairs that cause pronounced pain and irritation to the skin. Heating or drying the herb eliminates this problem.

PEPPERMINT *(Mentha × piperita)*

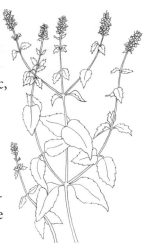

Parts used: Aerial parts.

Actions: Carminative, anti-inflammatory, anti-spasmodic, aromatic, diaphoretic, anti-emetic, nervine, antimicrobial, analgesic.

Indications: Peppermint is an excellent carminative because it relaxes the muscles of the digestive system. It combats flatulence and stimulates the flow of bile and digestive juices. It is used to relieve intestinal colic, flatulent dyspepsia, and associated conditions. The volatile oil acts as a mild anesthetic to the stomach wall and helps relieve feelings of nausea. It's commonly used to relieve nausea and vomiting related to pregnancy or traveling.

Peppermint can be used to treat ulcerative conditions of the bowels. Traditionally, it's been used to treat fever, colds, and the flu. Used as an inhalant, it provides temporary relief from nasal catarrh. It may be helpful for headaches associated with digestive problems. As a nervine, it eases anxiety and tension. It's also helpful for treating painful menstrual periods. Externally, peppermint is used to relieve itching and inflammation.

Preparation and Dosage: To make an infusion, pour 1 cup (240 ml) boiling water over 1 heaping teaspoon dried herb; let infuse 10 minutes. Drink as often as necessary.

When using a tincture, take 1–2 ml three times a day.

PLEURISY ROOT (Asclepias tuberosa)

Part used: Root.

Actions: Diaphoretic, expectorant, antispasmodic, carminative, anti-inflammatory.

Indications: Pleurisy root is an effective remedy for respiratory infections because it reduces inflammations and helps expectoration. It can be used to treat bronchitis and other chest conditions. It also has diaphoretic and antispasmodic powers, making it highly valued for treating pleurisy, pneumonia, and the flu.

Preparation and Dosage: To make an infusion, pour 1 cup (240 ml) boiling water over ½–1 teaspoon herb; let infuse 10–15 minutes. Drink three times a day.

When using a tincture, take 1–2 ml three times a day.

Contraindications: Do not use pleurisy root during pregnancy. Fresh pleurisy root may cause nausea and vomiting.

RED CLOVER *(Trifolium pratense)*

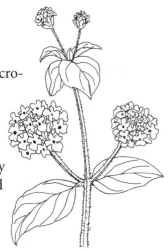

Part used: Flower heads.
Actions: Alterative, expectorant, antispasmodic.
Indications: Red clover is one of the most useful remedies for children with skin problems. It may be used safely for any case of childhood eczema. It's also valuable in the treatment of other chronic skin conditions, such as psoriasis.

Red clover is most useful for children but is also useful for adults. Because of its expectorant and antispasmodic actions, it has a role in the treatment of coughs and bronchitis. It's especially good for whooping cough.
Preparation and Dosage: To make an infusion, pour 1 cup (240 ml) boiling water over 1–3 teaspoons dried herb; let infuse 10–15 minutes. Drink three times a day.

When using a tincture, take 2–6 ml three times a day.
Contraindications: Red clover shoud not be used by pregnant women or people taking blood-thinning agents.

SAGE *(Salvia officinalis)*

Part used: Leaves.
Actions: Carminative, antispasmodic, antimicrobial, astringent, anti-inflammatory.
Indications: Sage is the classic remedy for inflammations of the mouth, throat, and tonsils because its volatile oils soothe mucous membranes. It may be used internally and as a mouthwash for treating inflamed and bleeding gums (gingivitis), inflamed tongue (glossitis), or generalized mouth inflammation (stomatitis). It's an excellent remedy for mouth ulcers (aphthae).

As a gargle, sage aids in the treatment of laryngitis, pharyngitis, tonsillitis, and quinsy. It's a valuable carminative that's often used for treating indigestion. It reduces sweating when taken internally, and it may be used to reduce the production of breast milk. As a compress, it promotes healing of wounds. Because sage stimulates the muscles of the uterus, it shouldn't be used during pregnancy.

Preparation and Dosage: To make an infusion, pour 1 cup (240 ml) boiling water over 1–2 teaspoons leaves; let infuse 10 minutes. Drink three times a day.

When making a mouthwash, put 2 teaspoons leaves in 1 pint (500 ml) water. Bring to a boil and let stand, covered, for 15 minutes. Gargle deeply with the hot tea for 5–10 minutes several times a day.

When using a tincture, take 2–4 ml three times a day.

Contraindications: Do not use sage during pregnancy.

SENECA SNAKEROOT *(Polygala senega)*

Part used: Root.

Actions: Expectorant, diaphoretic, sialogogue, emetic.

Indications: Seneca snakeroot comes to us from the Seneca nation of Native Americans, who used it for many problems, including snakebite. It has excellent expectorant effects that are helpful for treating bronchitic asthma, especially when expectoration is difficult. It may be used as a mouthwash and gargle in the treatment of pharyngitis and laryngitis, but excessive use irritates the lining of the gut and can lead to vomiting.

Preparation and Dosage: To make an infusion, pour 1 cup (240 ml) boiling water over ½ teaspoon dried root; let infuse 5–10 minutes. Drink 1 cup (240 ml) three times a day.

When using a tincture, take 1–2 ml three times a day.

SKUNK CABBAGE (*Symplocarpus foetidus*)

Parts used: Root and rhizome, dried.
Actions: Antispasmodic, diaphoretic, expectorant.
Indications: Skunk cabbage may be used whenever the lungs are experiencing tension or spasms. It helps relax and ease irritable coughs. It may be used for asthma, bronchitis, and whooping cough. As a diaphoretic, it aids the body during fevers.
Preparation and Dosage: Skunk cabbage is ordinarily used as a powder. Add 1 part powdered dried herb to 8 parts honey. Take ½–1 teaspoon of the mixture three times a day.

To make an infusion, pour 1 cup (240 ml) boiling water over ½ teaspoon (2 ml) herb; let stand, then drink.

When using a tincture, take ½–1 ml three times a day.
Contraindications: Skunk cabbage contains oxylate. It is not for long-term use or use by people with kidney disease.

SUNDEW (*Drosera rotundifolia*)

Part used: Entire plant.
Actions: Antispasmodic, demulcent, expectorant.
Indications: Sundew is helpful for treating bronchitis and whooping cough. It contains plumbagin, which seems active against *Streptococcus, Staphylococcus,* and *Pneumococcus* species. In fact, sundew can help with infections throughout the respiratory system.

Sundew has a relaxing effect on involuntary muscles, and this makes it useful for relieving asthma. In addition to having pulmonary effects, it has a long history of use in the treatment of stomach ulcers.
Preparation and Dosage: To make an infusion, pour 1 cup (240 ml) boiling water over 1 teaspoon dried herb; let infuse 10–15 minutes. Drink three times a day.

When using a tincture, take 1–2 ml three times a day.

SWEET VIOLET *(Viola odorata)*

Parts used: Leaves and flowers.
Actions: Expectorant, alterative, anti-inflammatory, diuretic.
Indications: Sweet violet has a long history of use as a cough remedy and is especially helpful for the treatment of bronchitis. It also may be used to help treat upper respiratory catarrh. Sweet violet is sometimes used for skin conditions like eczema and has been used to relieve rheumatism. It may be used for urinary infections and has a reputation as an anticancer herb. Regardless of whether this is true, sweet violet definitely has a role in holistic approaches to cancer treatment.
Preparation and Dosage: To make an infusion, pour 1 cup (240 ml) boiling water over 1 teaspoon herb; let infuse 10–15 minutes. Drink three times a day.

When using a tincture, take 1–2 ml three times a day.

THYME *(Thymus vulgaris)*

Parts used: Leaves, flowering tops.
Actions: Carminative, antimicrobial, antispasmodic, expectorant, astringent, anthelmintic.
Indications: Thyme contains large amounts of volatile oils and is therefore an effective carminative for dyspepsia and sluggish digestion. The oil is very antiseptic, and this explains why thyme can be used externally as a lotion for infected wounds. Internally, it helps with respiratory and digestive infections. It can be used as a gargle for laryngitis, tonsillitis, sore throat, and irritable coughs. It's an excellent cough remedy, producing expectoration and reducing unnecessary spasms. It may be used for bronchitis,

whooping cough, and asthma. As a gentle astringent, it has also been used for childhood diarrhea and bedwetting.

Preparation and Dosage: To make an infusion, pour 1 cup (240 ml) boiling water over 2 teaspoons dried herb; let infuse 10 minutes. Drink three times a day.

When using a tincture, take 2–4 ml three times a day.

WILD CHERRY BARK *(Prunus serotina)*

Part used: Bark, dried.

Actions: Antitussive, expectorant, astringent, nervine, antispasmodic.

Indications: Because of its powerful sedative action on the cough reflex, wild cherry bark is mainly used to treat irritating coughs; it's often used for bronchitis or whooping cough. (It's important to remember, however, that relieving a cough does not mean that you have taken care of underlying infections.) Wild cherry bark is helpful in controlling asthma. It may also be used as a bitter when digestion is sluggish. A cold infusion made from the bark may be helpful as a wash for inflamed eyes.

Preparation and Dosage: To make an infusion, pour 1 cup (240 ml) boiling water over 1 teaspoon dried bark; let infuse 10–15 minutes. Drink three times a day.

When using a tincture, take 1–2 ml three times a day.

Contraindications: Avoid long-term use of wild cherry bark.

WILD INDIGO *(Baptisia tinctoria)*

Part used: Root.

Actions: Antimicrobial, anticatarrhal.

Indications: Wild indigo should be considered for all infections that are focused in the respiratory system. It's especially useful in the treatment of infections and catarrh in the ear, nose, and throat. It may be used for laryngitis, tonsillitis, pharyngitis, and catarrhal infections of the nose and sinuses. When taken internally or used as a mouthwash, it helps heal mouth ulcers and gingivitis and control pyorrhea.

As a systemic remedy, it may be helpful in the treatment of enlarged and inflamed lymph glands (lymphadenitis) and in the reduction of fever. Externally, an ointment containing this herb helps with infected ulcers and sore nipples. When used as a douche, a wild indigo decoction helps relieve leukorrhea.

Preparation and Dosage: To make a decoction, put ½–1 teaspoon dried root in 1 cup water (240 ml). Bring to a boil and let simmer 10–15 minutes. Drink three times a day.

When using a tincture, take 1 ml three times a day.

YARROW *(Achillea millefolium)*

Parts used: Aerial parts.

Actions: Diaphoretic, hypotensive, astringent, anti-inflammatory, diuretic, antimicrobial, bitter, hepatic.

Indications: Yarrow, one of the best diaphoretic herbs, is a standard remedy for fever. It lowers blood pressure by dilating the peripheral vessels, and it stimulates digestion and tones the blood vessels. As a urinary antiseptic, it is indicated for infections like cystitis. Used externally, it aids in the healing of wounds. It's specifically indicated in thrombotic conditions associated with hypertension.

Preparation and Dosage: To make an infusion, pour 1 cup (240 ml) boiling water over 1–2 teaspoons dried herb; let infuse 10–15 minutes. Drink hot three times a day. When feverish, drink hourly.

When using a tincture, take 2–4 ml three times a day.

Contraindications: Do not use yarrow during pregnancy. Do not use over long periods of time.

6

MAKING
HERBAL MEDICINE

There is nothing mysterious about making healing formulations from plants, and it doesn't require any particular talent. The pharmaceutical elite would like us to think that to be of any use, a medicine must be made by a Pharm.D. wearing a white lab coat and must be packaged with half an acre of rainforest material. Not so! If you can make a cup of tea and cook a meal that your friends would be willing to eat, you are qualified.

Various methods for using plants have developed over the centuries. Our ancestors probably first used herbs by eating the fresh plant. Since then, over the thousands of years in which herbs have been used, other methods of preparing them have been developed. With our modern knowledge of pharmacology, we can consciously choose the best process for releasing the biochemical constituents that are all-important to healing — without insulting the integrity of the plant by isolating fractions of the whole.

The most effective way to use herbs is to take them internally, since healing takes place from within. Internal remedies can be prepared in many ways, but you should always approach the process with care to be sure that you get the desired result.

TEAS

Water-based teas can be made as *infusions* and *decoctions.* There are some basic rules for choosing which method to use with what herb, but, of course, there are many exceptions.

Infusions and Decoctions

Infusions are appropriate for nonwoody materials, such as leaves, flowers, and some stems. Decoctions are necessary if the herb contains any hard or woody material, like roots, barks, or nuts. The denser the plant or individual cell walls, the more energy is needed to extract cell content into the tea. This is where decocting comes into play.

As with anything in the real world, not every herb falls neatly into a category. This is especially true of roots that are rich in volatile oil, such as valerian root. The woodiness of the root suggests decocting, but if the roots are simmered, the therapeutically important volatile oil boils off.

Making an Infusion

If you know how to make tea, you know how to make an infusion. Infusions are best for the nonwoody parts of a plant, in which the active ingredients are easily accessible. Bark, root, seeds, or resin should be powdered first to break down some of the cell walls; this makes them more accessible to water. Seeds, such as fennel and aniseed, should be slightly bruised before infusion to release the volatile oils from the cells. Any aromatic herb should be infused in a well-sealed pot to ensure that only a minimum of the volatile oil is lost through evaporation.

An infusion is the simplest way to use fresh and dried herbs. However, fresh and dried herbs differ in water content. One part dried herb is equivalent to 3 parts fresh herb. For instance, if a recipe calls for 1 teaspoon of dried herb, substitute 3 teaspoons of fresh herb.

HOW TO MAKE AN INFUSION

Step 1. In a china or glass teapot that has been warmed, add about 1 teaspoon dried herb for each cup of tea.

Step 2. Pour in 1 cup (240 ml) boiling water for each teaspoon of herb and put the lid on the teapot. Steep 10 to 15 minutes.

Step 3. Strain the tea while still hot, and drink.

Making Large and Cold Infusions

It's usually best to drink medicinal herb teas hot, but infusions can also be drunk cold. If the herbs are sensitive to heat because they contain highly volatile oils or because their constituents break down at high temperatures, make a cold infusion. The proportion of herb to water is the same, but the herb should be left to infuse for 6 to 12 hours in a well-sealed pot of cool water. When ready, strain and drink. Infusions can be sweetened to taste. If you prefer to avoid the messiness of loose leaves, make tea bags by filling small muslin bags with herbal mixtures, taking care to remember how many teaspoons have been put in each bag. Use these tea bags just as you would use ordinary tea bags.

Larger quantities of infusions can be made in the proportion of 1 ounce (30 g) of herb to 1 pint (500 ml) of water. It's best to store leftovers in the refrigerator because their shelf life is short; any microorganism that enters the infusion will multiply and thrive in it. If there is any sign of fermentation or spoilage, the infusion should be discarded. Whenever possible, infusions should be freshly prepared.

The Best Herbs for Infusions

Many herbal infusions are exquisite additions to our lifestyles and can open up a whole world of subtle delights and pleasures.

They are not only medicines or "alternatives" to coffee but can be excellent beverages in their own right. Everyone will discover his or her own preferred herbs, but here are some of my favorites. They may be used singly or in combination, and selection can be based on both taste and medicinal properties.

- **Flowers:** chamomile, elderflower, hibiscus, linden blossom, red clover
- **Leaves:** peppermint, spearmint, lemon balm, rosemary, lemon verbena
- **Berries:** hawthorn, rose hips
- **Seeds:** aniseed, caraway, celery, dill, fennel
- **Roots:** licorice

Making a Decoction

If the herbs you've selected are hard and woody, a decoction — which requires more heat than an infusion — will ensure that the soluble contents of the herbs actually reach the water. Roots, rhizomes, wood, bark, nuts, and some seeds are hard and have very strong cell walls, and decoctions are suitable for these materials.

HOW TO MAKE A DECOCTION

Step 1. In a glass, ceramic, earthenware, or enameled metal pot or saucepan, put 1 teaspoon dried herb for each cup (240 ml) water. If larger quantities are desired, use 1 ounce (30 g) dried herb for each pint (500 ml) water.

Step 2. Add a cup (240 ml) water for each teaspoon dried herb. Bring to a boil and simmer for 10 to 15 minutes or the amount of time specified for the particular herb or mixture. If the herb contains volatile oils, put a lid on the pot.

Step 3. Strain the tea while still hot, and drink.

If you're preparing a mixture that contains both soft and woody herbs, prepare separate infusions and decoctions to ensure that the more sensitive herbs are treated properly. Combine the two liquids and drink.

TINCTURES

Extracts of herbs in alcohol or glycerin are called *tinctures*. Because tinctures are much stronger, volume for volume, than infusions or decoctions, the dose taken is usually much smaller. Tinctures may be used in various ways. They can be taken straight or can be mixed with water. If a tincture is added to hot water, the alcohol in the tincture will largely evaporate, leaving most of the extract in the water. A few drops of tincture can also be added to a bath or foot bath, used in a compress, or mixed with oil and fat to make an ointment. Suppositories and lozenges can also be made from tinctures.

Alcohol is a better solvent than water for most plant constituents because it dissolves nearly all of the ingredients and acts as a preservative. Tinctures with a glycerin base have the advantage of being milder on the digestive tract. However, glycerin does not dissolve resinous or oily materials well. As a solvent, glycerin is generally better than water but not as good as alcohol.

How to Make a Tincture

The method outlined here is a basic approach. Remember, if you are using fresh rather than dried herbs, use twice the amount.

Step 1. In a container that can be tightly closed, place 4 ounces (120 g) finely chopped or ground dried herb. Pour 1 pint (500 ml) 60-proof vodka over the herbs and close the container tightly with a lid.

Step 2. Place the container in a warm, dark place for 2 weeks and shake it once a day.

Step 3. Strain the liquid through a muslin cloth suspended in a bowl. Wring out all the liquid from the herbs. (The spent herbs make excellent compost!)

Step 4. Pour the tincture into a dark bottle. It should be labeled and kept tightly closed.

Other Tincture Bases

Tinctures can also be made in a glycerin base, which is milder on the digestive tract and doesn't involve other problems associated with alcohol. However, the disadvantage is that glycerin does not dissolve resinous or oily plant material well. As a solvent, glycerin is generally better than water but not as good as alcohol. If using glycerin as the solvent, mix H pint (250 ml) glycerin and ½ pint (250 ml) water (for fresh herbs, use a mixture of 75 percent glycerin to 25 percent water). Pour this mixture over the herbs and close container tightly with a lid. Another way to make a kind of alcohol tincture is to infuse herbs in wine. Wine-based preparations do not have the shelf life of other tinctures and are less concentrated, but they can be both pleasant to take and effective.

DRY HERB PREPARATIONS

There are many advantages to taking herbs in a dry form; the main one is that the taste of the herb can be avoided while the whole herb (including the woody material) is consumed. Unfortunately, the practice of taking dry herbs also has a number of drawbacks.

- Dry herbs are unprocessed, so the constituents are not always readily available for absorption. In an infusion, heat and water help to break down the walls of the plant cells and dissolve the constituents. The digestive process of the stomach and small intestines, in contrast, is not guaranteed to break down plant cell walls.

- When plant constituents are already dissolved in liquid form, they are available much faster and begin their action sooner.
- Bitter herbs work best when tasted because their effects result from a neurologic reflex. When bitters are put into a capsule or pill, their actions may be lost or diminished.

Given all of these considerations, there are several ways to use herbs in dry form. Always be sure that the herbs are powdered as finely as possible. Grinding guarantees that the cell walls are largely broken down and helps in digestion and absorption.

Capsules

It's convenient to use powdered herbs in gelatin capsules. The necessary capsule size depends on the amount of herbs prescribed per dose, the density of the plant, and the volume of the material. A size "00" capsule, for instance, holds about ⅙ ounce (5 g) of finely powdered herb.

MAKING YOUR OWN CAPSULES

Filling a capsule is easy. You can find the empty capsule containers (size "00") for sale at a health food store.

Step 1. Place the powdered herbs on a flat dish and separate the halves of the capsule.

Step 2. Move the halves of the capsule through the powder, scooping the herb into the two halves.

Step 3. Push the halves of the capsule together.

Pills

Pills can be made in many ways, some very simple and some complex. The simplest way to take an unpleasant remedy is to roll the powder into a small ball with fresh bread. This works most effectively with strong-tasting herbs such as goldenseal or cayenne.

RESOURCES

NHLBI Information Center
P.O. Box 30105
Bethesda, MD 20824-0105
Telephone: (301) 251-1222
Web site: www.nhlbi.nih.gov/nhlbi/nhlbi.htm

This center is a service of the National Heart, Lung, and Blood Institute (NHLBI) of the National Institutes of Health and provides information to health professionals, patients, and the public about the treatment, diagnosis, and prevention of heart, lung, and blood diseases.

Office on Smoking and Health,
Public Information Branch
4770 Buford Highway NE.
Mail Stop K50
Atlanta, GA 30341-3724
Telephone: (404) 488-5705

Information about smoking and health.

INDEX

Entries in **bold** indicate recipes; page references in *italics* indicate illustrations.

OTHER BOOKS IN THE STOREY MEDICINAL HERB GUIDE SERIES

Healthy Heart, by David Hoffmann. 128 pages. Paperback. ISBN 1-58017-251-2.

Healthy Digestion, by David Hoffmann. 128 pages. Paperback. ISBN 1-58017-250-4.

Healthy Bones and Joints, by David Hoffmann. 128 pages. Paperback. ISBN 1-58017-253-9.

Herbs for Hepatitis C and the Liver, by Stephen Harrod Buhner. 128 pages. Paperback. ISBN 1-58017-255-5.

Herbal Antibiotics, by Stephen Harrod Buhner. 128 pages. Paperback. ISBN 1-58017-148-6.

Dandelion Medicine, by Brigitte Mars. 128 pages. Paperback. ISBN 1-58017-207-5.

Saw Palmetto for Men and Women, by David Winston. 128 pages. Paperback. ISBN 1-58017-206-7.

Natural First Aid, by Brigitte Mars. 128 pages. Paperback. ISBN 1-58017-147-8.

ADHD Alternatives, by Aviva Romm and Tracy Romm. 128 pages. Paperback. ISBN 1-58017-248-2.

These books and other Storey books are available at your bookstore, farm store, garden center, or directly from Storey Books, Schoolhouse Road, Pownal, Vermont 05261, or by calling 1-800-441-5700. Or visit our Web site at www.storeybooks.com.